OVERCOMING
MIGRAINE

OVERCOMING MIGRAINE

A Proven Plan for Prevention

LYNN H. CLAYTON, RD, LDN

OVERCOMING MIGRAINE

ISBN: 978-1-7352679-1-3 (paperback)

ISBN: 978-1-7352679-0-6 (Kindle)

Get Your FREE Overcoming Migraine Prevention Plan

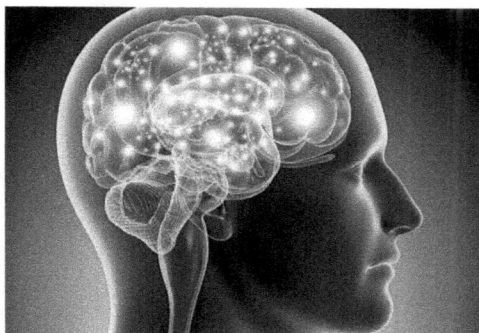

To say thank you for buying my book, I would like to give you your own **Migraine Prevention Plan.**

Take the quiz and get details to create your personalized migraine prevention plan.

To Download Go To:

https://ourdailychews.com/ overcoming-migraine-prevention-plan/

Contents

Introduction

IF YOU HAVE MIGRAINE headaches or think you may have migraines, this book is for you. If you know someone battling migraines, this is the book to share with them. Anyone suffering the debilitating effects of a migraine will gladly welcome help to avoid having another one. Once you have experienced a migraine headache, you know almost immediately when another one starts to come on. The fear of experiencing another migraine can become almost as tortuous as the pain itself. Imagine what your life would be like if you no longer had to suffer from migraines. What would you be able to accomplish? What would you feel free to do? How would you spend your time? What would you spend your money on if you were not spending it on medication or trips to the emergency room?

Fortunately for migraine sufferers, research in recent years is leading to a better understanding of the pathophysiology, or cause, of migraine and possible treatments. Unfortunately, the research takes a while to catch up with the medical community, so many sufferers do not find the relief they are seeking. My goal is to help you understand your body and the mechanisms by which migraine occurs. If you can incorporate a few changes into your lifestyle, you can greatly reduce the impact of this painful disease on your life. In this book, we will define migraine, discuss current theories on causes, explore triggers (including a chapter on diet) and discuss prevention and treatment options.

INTRODUCTION

As a migraine sufferer for over three decades, my goal is to offer you a practical explanation of migraine as we understand it today. You will learn perhaps more than you ever wanted to know about migraine. But I hope you gain some insight into what causes or contributes to your migraines. Prevention and treatment options will be discussed in chapters 5 and 7 with chapter 6 taking an in-depth look at diet. It takes a little work and some effort, but you can regain control of your life without constant fear of another migraine lurking around the corner. This book includes information that I wish I had known years ago. It took decades of trial and error and educating myself to learn what works and what does not. I want to offer you hope for a brighter future. So, dive in and take charge of those headaches so you can get back to living life.

To Good Health (and fewer migraines)!

SECTION 1

Migraines:
What Are They and
What Causes Them?

— 1 —
Explaining Migraine

History of Migraine

MIGRAINES HAVE PLAGUED sufferers for thousands of years. They are one of the oldest ailments known to mankind. Migraine headaches were first recorded around 3,000 B.C. during the Mesopotamian Era.[1] The ancient Egyptians recorded cases of headache with neuralgia (nerve pain) as early as 1200 BC. Hippocrates, considered the father of modern medicine, described the visual disturbances that can occur prior to these headaches as early as 400 BC. Aretaeus of Cappadocia, an ancient Greek physician, is credited as the discoverer of migraines. In the second century, he described symptoms of attacks of a unilateral headache associated with vomiting. The first known use of the term for this headache was in the 15th century by Galen of Pergamum, who was a Greek physician, writer, and philosopher. He used the Latin word "hemicrania"—meaning half (hemi) and skull (crania)—to describe the pain occurring on one side of the head during an attack. The word was later translated to French, which is where we get the word *migraine*.[2]

Even before these horrible headaches were named, the treatments abounded for *migraineurs* (people who suffer from migraines). Ancient treatments date as far back as 3,000 BC and included trepanation (drilling a hole in the skull to release evil spirits), bloodletting, applying a hot iron to the site of pain, and inserting a clove of garlic through an incision made in the temple.[3] Interventions were based on medical knowledge of the time or superstitious beliefs. As you can imagine, the treatments were not pleasant or without risk and some died from infection.

What is Migraine?

Migraine is more than just a headache! Unlike tension headaches, migraines involve a complex neurological process which can include symptoms such as visual or auditory disturbances; sensitivity to light, sound, smells or touch; nausea and vomiting; tingling or numbness in extremities and involuntary muscle movement. Neurological symptoms are typically accompanied by head pain but not always. A "usual" migraine headache occurs suddenly, presents as moderate to severe throbbing pain on one side of the head, lasts longer than six hours and may last several days with varying levels of pain.[4] There is typically a recovery period following the symptoms where you may feel fatigue, have a stiff neck, be sensitive to light or sound and even have a dull headache. This is what I refer to as a migraine hangover. These symptoms gradually resolve and there will be headache-free periods between migraines.

Diagnosing Migraine

There is no test for migraine. They do not show up on computed topography (CT) scans or magnetic resonance imaging (MRI) or in bloodwork, however, your doctor may order these tests to rule out possible causes of headache and neurological symptoms such as infection, aneurysm, or tumors.[5] If other life-threatening conditions are ruled out, your doctor will rely on symptoms for diagnosis. Providing your doctor with a complete health history and symptom log is the quickest (and least expensive) way to get a proper diagnosis. Migraine can manifest in different ways. It is important to give your doctor details so he or she can determine if you have migraines, what type of migraine you have and how best to treat it.

According to the International Classification of Headache Disorders (ICHD), migraines are a primary headache (not caused by another condition) as opposed to a secondary headache (caused by another condition such as trauma or a brain tumor). Migraines are divided into types or categories based on *symptoms or frequency.* I will discuss both types in more detail.

Types of Migraine

Migraines classified based on symptoms are divided into *migraine with aura* and *migraine without aura.* An *aura* is a group of neurological symptoms that signal the beginning of a migraine and usually affect vision causing temporary blind spots, blurry vision or tunnel vision, flashing lights or zigzag lines and may or may not involve eye pain. Head pain can begin within a few minutes after the onset of the aura or several hours later. A headache does not always follow an aura. Only about 25% of migraine sufferers experience an aura.[6] Symptoms of either type can include a throbbing pain typically on one side of the head, nausea, vomiting, sensitivity to light, sound or odors, and numbness or tingling sensations. Migraines generally last from 4 to 72 hours.[7]

Migraine can be further divided based on frequency. Migraines can be *acute* or episodic (only occurring occasionally) or *chronic* (occurring several days each month).

Classification of Migraine

According to the ICHD-3 Diagnosis Code, there are six diagnosis codes your doctor can use to classify migraine and associated disorders. There are thirteen other classifications for headache listed besides migraine. Four of these are considered primary headache and the other ten involve secondary headaches stemming from another condition such as infection, trauma, or tumor. It is possible to experience more than one type and people with migraines often experience other types of headaches.

The purpose of this book is to address migraine as a primary condition. If migraines are caused by another condition, then that condition should be addressed and corrected or treated first to avoid migraine as a secondary headache.

Treating Migraine

Not every disease is best treated by drugs, and migraine is no exception. Pharmaceutical drugs have their place and are sometimes necessary and much appreciated. But relying exclusively on a pill to fix a problem will not get you best results. Their purpose is to address symptoms by blocking pain receptors, affecting neurotransmitters like serotonin, or working on blood vessels surrounding the brain. While this can provide relief in some cases, it does not address the underlying cause of those symptoms. While there is still more to be learned about migraine, we can use the knowledge already available to make positive changes and improve your life as a migraine sufferer. In this book we will look at ways to balance serotonin and hormones thought to be involved in migraine. We will identify dietary components linked to migraine occurrence and discuss importance of getting adequate nutrients from our diet or supplements. And of course, we cannot overlook lifestyle factors such as stress management, sleep quality and quantity, and environmental influences.

Statistics

Several famous people in history have suffered from migraine headaches. These include Julius Caesar, Napoleon Bonaparte, Charles Darwin, Sigmund Freud, Vincent Van Gough, Albert Einstein, Thomas Jefferson, John F. Kennedy and Elvis Presley to name a few.[8] In fact, according to the Migraine Research Foundation, about 39 million Americans and 1 billion men, women and children worldwide suffer from migraine headaches. Migraine is the third most prevalent disease in the world behind dental caries and tension-type headaches, and the leading cause of disability among all neurological disorders.[9] About 18% of American women, 6% of men, and 10% of children experience migraines.[10]

Migraine tends to run in families. About 90% of migraine sufferers have a family history of migraine according to the Migraine Research Foundation. Migraines are one of the most common complaints neurologists treat in daily practice. It has taken several centuries and a few different theories, but scientists are getting closer to revealing the true cause and mechanism involved in migraine headaches. That is fortunate for us, so no one else must endure those archaic treatments of times past.

— 2 —
Causes of Migraine

To TREAT ANY condition, we must first know the cause. Migraines are no exception. If we can determine the cause of migraine, then we can plan accordingly to prevent or at least control migraines. And by controlling migraines, I mean reducing the intensity and frequency with which they occur. Currently, the exact cause of migraine is unknown, but there are a few theories which have led to potentially helpful treatments. In this chapter, we will look at risk factors for migraine, what occurs in the brain during a migraine attack and the stages of a migraine.

Risk Factors for Migraine

Your risk for getting migraines is affected by three factors that predispose you to developing migraines at some point in your life. You may have one or all three. The three risk factors for migraine are:

1. **Genetics** – For years, researchers suspected that genes play a role in the development of migraine because a family history of migraine increases your risk. Migraines are inherited in 60–80% of cases.[1] Scientists have discovered gene variations that may increase the risk of migraine.[2] However, having a genetic variation does not mean

you will inevitably get migraines. Scientists believe migraine is a complex disease in which multiple genetic variations contribute to the underlying risk, with each variation having a relatively small effect. Even though genetic variants may be involved, they are neither necessary nor sufficient to cause migraine. Migraine susceptibility is rather a result of the interaction of genetic variations with each other and with environmental and lifestyle factors.

2. **Gender** – Females are three times more likely to have migraines than males according to the *Office of Women's Health*. This is thought to be due to hormonal changes in women associated with menstruation, pregnancy, and menopause. Women may notice more migraines surrounding their period. Some may notice that migraines get worse or get better during pregnancy. Hormone changes during the menopausal stage may also change migraine patterns. After menopause, migraines tend to lessen or stop completely.[3]

3. **Certain medical conditions** – Having certain health conditions can increase your risk of migraines. These include anxiety, depression, bipolar disorder, sleep disorder and epilepsy.[4] There are other conditions with a possible connection to migraine, but more research is needed to discover the connection. Some people may start experiencing migraines as a result of head trauma, neck issues, or Chiari malformation (a condition where part of the brain tissue extends into the spinal column). In these instances, migraines are a secondary headache caused by another condition.

Pathophysiology of Migraines – What Happens During a Migraine

Medical research continues to improve our understanding of what may happen before and during a migraine attack. Many theories regarding the cause of migraine have been proposed over the centuries. One theory proposes that changes in blood vessels surrounding the brain cause the pain associated with migraines. These changes produce *vasoconstriction* (narrowing of blood vessels) followed by *vasodilation* (widening of blood vessels). This theory was originally noted in the fifteenth century by Galen of Pergamum.[5] The theory was supported by the fact that some migraines are helped by taking medication that acts on blood vessels. In the late 1930s, Harold Wolff and John Graham discovered the drug *ergotamine* could provide relief for migraines.[6] Ergotamine works by narrowing the blood vessels around the brain. Since blood vessels around the brain are surrounded by sensitive nerve fibers, changes in blood vessel diameter may explain the excruciating pain associated with migraines. But what causes this change in the diameter of blood vessels? Why does this occur in some people and not others? It is also interesting to note here that the brain has no sensory (pain) receptors and therefore does not feel pain itself. That is why neurosurgeons can perform surgery on a brain while the person is wide awake. But the brain is our processing center for pain, meaning that it interprets pain signals from the rest of our body, including the structures surrounding the brain itself.

More recent research shows that changes in blood vessel diameter are not always present during migraine. Alternatively, changes in blood vessels do not always cause migraine.[7] Even when blood vessel changes are associated with migraine, it does not explain the cause of those changes. Researchers now believe migraine is neurological in origin. Recent research shows evidence that changes occurring before the onset of a migraine are *neurogenic* (caused by the nervous system) and may be associated with malfunction of neurotransmitters, particularly serotonin, in the brain. It is thought that this neurological reaction can trigger changes in blood vessels. The neurological component explains the associated symptoms, especially in migraines with aura, which include visual disturbances, numbness, tingling and mood changes. Most experts believe that this may be caused by a phenomenon in the brain called *cortical spreading depression* (CSD).[8] CSD can be described as seizure-like activity in the brain, caused by hyperactive neurons, followed by a period of suppressed neuron activity. This phenomenon produces neurological changes in the brain that may affect mood, perception of sights, sounds and smells as well as changes in appetite. During a migraine, this excitability occurs as a slow wave of activity spreading across the cortical area of the brain causing numerous physiological changes that include release of neurotransmitters, changes in blood flow, and a decrease in oxygen.[9] The time it takes for this wave to move from one area to another varies and implies that it is mediated by a chemical substance. Science has not yet identified the chemical involved. To visualize what occurs, imagine a small rock tossed into a pond. The ripple effect represents the slow wave of activity as it spreads out across the water. Once the ripples disappear, the effect of the rock has subsided. In the brain, this can take hours or even days and corresponds to the duration of a migraine. CSD is thought to be the underlying cause of aura but whether it directly contributes to headache is less clear. Although a headache usually follows aura, the headache is thought to occur due to activation of pain receptors via release of proinflammatory vasodilators by the trigeminal nerve. The trigeminal nerve, also known as the fifth cranial nerve, provides nerve sensation to the meninges, which are the three membranes that surround the brain. Due to the neurological changes that occur, it is possible that CSD indirectly activates the trigeminal nerve. This appears to be the final event leading to pain of migraine.

Finding the origin of this reaction is complicated. Nerves can act on blood vessels, but blood vessels can also release chemicals that affect nerves. Endothelial cells of the blood vessels can release inflammatory immune cells in response to potential threats. Any chemical, mechanical or thermal stimuli could be perceived as a threat. This perceived threat triggers the release of chemicals which launch an immune response for defense. During activation of the immune response, changes occur that may trigger migraine in susceptible individuals. For those without migraine, this sensory stimulation in the cortical region would go undetected.

Another contributor in the process is the release of serotonin by circulating platelets (blood cells involved in clotting). Serotonin causes vasoconstriction (narrowing of blood vessels) which reduces blood flow and helps clots to form. This is helpful for wound healing. But what triggers the release of serotonin from platelets without the presence of a wound? The release of serotonin (as well as histamine) from platelets may be related to antigen–antibody reactions and may explain inflammation as a factor.[10]

The complexity of multiple factors involved in migraine makes it difficult to treat. Multiple approaches have been proposed based on what researchers have discovered so far. It will likely take a combination of therapy to successfully treat this complicated disease. We will discuss treatment options in chapters 7 and 8.

Stages of Migraine

Migraine tends to occur in stages. However, not every migraine will involve all four stages. Symptoms vary from person to person. The four stages of a migraine include **prodrome, aura, headache,** and **postdrome.**[11]

The **prodrome** occurs before the headache and may include sensitivity to light and sound, nausea, fatigue, dizziness, changes in appetite, neck pain or neck stiffness and mood changes. These physical and psychological changes can occur a few hours or a few days before a migraine headache manifests.

The second stage is the **aura.** For people who experience migraine with aura, the aura usually presents as a change in vision, such as seeing spots, flashing lights, zigzag lines or waves and may include blind spots or tunnel vision. The aura usually lasts about fifteen minutes but can persist for a few hours. While visual changes are the most common aura experienced, other symptoms may be present during the aura stage and include muscle weakness, hearing music or noises in your head that are not real, uncontrolled movements, confusion and difficulty speaking or understanding others. Since some of these symptoms may also be associated with a stroke, you may need testing to rule out more serious problems. Some people may get an aura without any other symptoms. This is called a silent migraine and tends to be more common in people over the age of 50.

The third stage of migraine is the **headache.** The headache is usually a throbbing pain occurring on one side of the head and is worse with movement. Nausea, vomiting, and sensitivity to light, sound and odors can be present.

Once the headache or other symptoms subside, you are in the **postdrome** phase. This phase may include fatigue, difficulty concentrating, weakness or dizziness. This last phase may be noticed immediately after a migraine and can persist for hours or a few days.

Stages of Migraine
1. Prodrome
2. Aura
3. Headache and associated symptoms
4. Postdrome

Can Migraine Increase Your Risk of Other Problems?

Migraine has been associated with a slight increased risk of stroke.[12] Migraine with aura has a slightly higher risk than without aura. Factors that can make this more likely include the use of birth control pills, hormone replacement therapy and smoking. Exercise, a healthy diet and maintaining a healthy weight can reduce the risk. If you experience stroke-like symptoms or an aura lasting more than an hour, seek medical help.

An association between migraine and seizures has been explored. It is possible that migraine can trigger a seizure and a seizure can trigger a migraine. People with seizure disorders are twice as likely to experience migraines.[13] This can lead to misdiagnosis since both have similar symptoms. If you experience seizure-like activity or lose consciousness during a migraine, talk to your doctor.

Other conditions that may be connected to migraine include heart disease, fibromyalgia and posttraumatic stress disorder (PTSD).[14] Research has yet to determine a common factor, and having migraine does not guarantee you will develop any of these. But it is good to be aware of, so you can make sure you are accurately diagnosed and treated.

Being prone to migraine does not mean you are doomed. Migraines need a trigger to initiate the process described earlier. Avoiding triggers will help prevent migraines from occurring. We will discuss possible triggers in chapter 3.

— 3 —
Triggers for Migraine

NOW THAT WE have discussed the possible causes of migraine, we will look at what may trigger the biochemical changes leading to migraine. Even if your genes, your gender and having certain health conditions predispose you to having migraines, that does not mean you will automatically develop migraines. Your diet, lifestyle and environment can either promote or prevent the internal changes leading to a migraine. Identifying and avoiding your migraine triggers plays an important role in preventing or reducing the frequency and intensity.

Scientists tell us that our health is based largely on lifestyle choices. Only about 20–30% of our health can be blamed on genetics. That means genes will only take you so far. Our environment and lifestyle choices affect how our genes are expressed. This is evident through the study of *epigenetics*. According to the *Oxford English Dictionary*, epigenetics is the study of changes in organisms caused by modification of gene expression rather than alteration of the genetic code itself. We are learning that certain healthy lifestyles seem to keep genes "turned off" or prevent them from expressing themselves so that disease does not manifest. I believe that may explain why some people with a genetic predisposition will never get migraines and why there are varying degrees of migraine. Migraine symptoms also present differently during different attacks, suggesting there are multiple factors involved. It is based not only on genes but on the factors that influence those genes. This is good news for all of us, regardless of the genes we inherit. While we cannot control our genes or our gender, we do have quite a bit of control when it comes to our health. Being aware of the impact our lifestyle choices have on our physiology goes a long way in controlling whether we trigger a migraine. In this chapter, we will focus on the factors most often implicated in triggering migraine.

Potential Migraine Triggers

There are several factors that influence our genes and biochemistry. We can divide these factors into dietary, lifestyle, and environmental. Once we learn which components trigger migraines, we are well on our way to taking charge of our health. We will briefly explore those factors here, and in section 2, we will discuss ways to modify them to help prevent or at least lessen the impact of migraine on our lives.

I have included triggers that seem to be common with migraines.[1] Several I have had personal experience with, as I will describe in the next chapter. You may notice that any one of these by itself does not always trigger a migraine. Some theorize that it may be a multifactorial event. If you have the right combination under the right circumstances, it can provoke a migraine. Keeping a headache log helps to determine which of these or which combination of these may trigger your migraines.

Dietary-Related Triggers

Dehydration

Allowing yourself to get dehydrated or even being mildly chronically dehydrated can lead to headaches including migraines. Drinking plenty of water or sugar-free, caffeine-free beverages throughout the day may help prevent or alleviate those annoying headaches.

Food triggers

Many migraine sufferers report some type of food trigger. These vary from one individual to the next and are best determined by keeping a diet diary along with a headache log. It may take time to determine which food or combination of foods are causing your migraines. Migraines do not always show up right after eating a food. It can manifest a few hours later or even the next day. Some common food triggers include chocolate, wine, aged cheese, and citrus fruit. If you have a food allergy or intolerance, you may notice a connection with that food and migraine, but it may not occur every time. Writing down what you eat takes some effort, but it may give you the information you need to change your diet to prevent migraines. We will cover food triggers in detail in chapter 6.

Fluctuations in blood sugar

A drop in blood sugar can cause a headache for anyone, but for those prone to migraines, it can be a trigger. Going too long between meals or skipping meals can cause a drop in blood sugar. Sudden increases in blood sugar from eating too much sugary foods followed by the inevitable crash or drop in blood sugar can be a trigger. Fasting or extreme dieting can also cause a drop in blood sugar. People with diabetes can experience headaches due to high or low blood sugar, which could potentially trigger migraines in susceptible individuals.

Lifestyle Factors

Sleep quality and quantity

Disrupted sleep cycles can trigger migraines. Changes such as not getting enough sleep or sleeping more than usual may throw off your body's normal rhythm making a migraine more likely to occur. People with sleep disorders are at risk of migraine.

Stress

Emotional, mental, or physical stress can all contribute to development of migraines. We know that people with anxiety, depression or bipolar disorder are more prone to migraines. But a person's ability to cope with stressors, such as work or family pressures, can impact their likelihood of developing a migraine. How we perceive stressors and how we react to them can be changed through learned behaviors and improved coping skills.

Physical activity

Vigorous activity can trigger migraine. Some people report onset of a migraine with sex. Everyone needs adequate exercise, but if you notice migraines after being physically active, try lower intensity workouts. Talk to your doctor if you have concerns about exercise-induced migraine.

Environmental Factors

Allergies

Certain scents (perfume, lotions, cigarette smoke) or seasonal allergies may trigger a histamine reaction which can trigger the cascade of events leading to a migraine.

Changes in the weather

Sudden changes in barometric pressure related to changes in weather such as thunderstorms may trigger a headache for some people. A change in seasons may also be a factor.

Light

Bright or flashing lights can trigger migraines. This may be due to stimulation of the brain leading to a hyperactive response in people sensitive to it.

Noise

Loud noises may trigger a migraine. This may be due to over stimulation as well.

Not every migraine sufferer will have the same triggers. It is important to keep track of those that seem to provoke a migraine for you.

Tips to Avoid Common Migraine Triggers

1. Watch what you eat and drink. Stay hydrated by getting adequate fluids (especially water) every day. Do not skip meals. Eat on a regular schedule to avoid fluctuations in blood sugar. If you get a headache, write down the foods and beverages you had before it started. Once you see a pattern, try avoiding those foods or beverages to see if your headaches improve.

2. Watch out for caffeine. Too much can cause migraines. But suddenly cutting out caffeine can cause headaches. If you are consuming a lot of caffeine, try slowly cutting back to see if your migraines improve.

3. Get regular sleep. If your sleep habits change or if you are allowing yourself to get overly tired, that can encourage onset of a migraine. Try getting 6–8 hours per night of quality sleep.

4. Be careful with exercise. Everyone needs regular physical activity, but too much exercise can trigger headaches for some people. If you notice more migraines after being physically active, talk to your doctor for modifications you can make in your exercise routine.

5. Downsize your stress. Exercise can be a great way to cope with stress. You may also try meditation, prayer, spending time with people you love, and doing things you enjoy. If you cannot avoid or change some of the things that make you tense, create a plan for dealing with that. Counseling and stress management classes can help. Learning to control your stress response through mindfulness, deep breathing and focused meditation may go a long way in preventing migraines.

6. Avoid environmental hazards. If you know certain scents, bright lights, or loud noises trigger migraine for you, develop a strategy to avoid those if possible. We cannot control weather changes, but you may be able to minimize the effects of other triggers so that weather changes do not bother you as much.

— 4 —
Personal Migraine Story

LOOKING AT MIGRAINES from a medical point of view is not the same as experiencing one yourself. Only another migraineur can sympathize or empathize with your pain. In this chapter, I will share my personal story that led me to research migraine headaches so I could understand how to relieve my own suffering.

It is possible that I experienced my first migraine headache in kindergarten. Kids can get migraines too. I remember one day when my head hurt so bad that I could not enjoy playing with my classmates. Even the activities were of no interest to me and all I felt like doing was laying my head on the desk and taking a nap, hoping the pain would stop. Since I was a shy kid, I did not say anything and tried to tough it out and pretend I was okay. Eventually, one of the teachers noticed that I was not my usual self. She asked me if I was okay to which I replied my head hurt and tears followed, to the best of my recollection. My mother was contacted, and she came to pick me up. As I waited for her to come, I felt relief that I was going home. My mom arrived and once we made it to the car, I threw up. I do not remember if the headache dissipated immediately after throwing up or not, but eventually, I felt better. There were no other symptoms that I recall. It was just a bad headache. Even though I had other headaches throughout my childhood, this one was memorable. It was years later before I experienced another migraine and eventually got a diagnosis.

It was a beautiful clear day in the spring of 1986. It was just another ordinary day at school. I had finished lunch and was enjoying some time outside with my high school classmates. The sun was bright and warm. We were happily exchanging autographs and words of wisdom in our yearbooks. As lunch time ended, we headed back inside to go to our next class. I remember my eyes having to adjust from the bright sunshine as we returned indoors. That was normal. But by the time I made it to my locker on the second floor, I knew something was not right. I was not seeing clearly. It seemed I had blind spots in my field of vision. It was a scary feeling. I did not know what it was, but something was wrong, so I headed to the school office. My mother was contacted and came to pick me up.

That afternoon I experienced the worst headache I had ever endured. As the pain grew worse, it felt as if my head would explode. I could not stand loud noises or bright light. Smells made me nauseous. I tried to find a comfortable position on the couch. Lying down made my head hurt worse and sitting up made me nauseous. The pain continued for what seemed like an eternity. Eventually, the nausea really set in and was followed by vomiting. Normally I hate to throw up, but the relief that I felt after removing the contents of my stomach made it worthwhile. As the headache finally subsided, I felt exhausted. What just happened? Would it happen again? I hoped not.

At the age of fifteen, that was my first true experience with a migraine. Nothing prepares you for that. I knew my mother had "bad headaches" occasionally, but I had never seen her in the shape I found myself in. Over the years, I learned more about migraines. But just because I understood migraines better, did not mean that I was okay with having more of them.

I had the genetic predisposition since my mother had migraines. My father also developed migraines in his forties. And my sister reported getting them during her college years. So, it appeared that my genes had doomed me to migraines. It is not likely that I will live the rest of my life without ever having another headache but with a few changes to my diet and lifestyle, I have greatly diminished the effect of headache on my life. I now enjoy months and occasionally an entire year migraine free. Other headaches like tension or sinus headaches may occasionally pop up, but they are no longer a normal part of my day.

I started to learn what triggered mine. That first migraine likely was provoked by the bright light from the sun reflecting off those white pages of the yearbook. Perhaps that combined with other factors, such as teenage hormones, what I had eaten for lunch or any stress I may have felt being in high school. Evidently that was enough to provoke my first attack of migraine. I had a few more during my teenage years. They were always scary, and the pain awful. But fortunately, my migraines only occurred several times a year. But when I had one, I was out of commission for the rest of the day.

My migraines became more frequent when I went to college. I moved to an apartment about an hour and a half away from home and enrolled in a dental hygiene program at a community college. My worst migraine occurred in my early twenties during my last year of dental hygiene school. My stress level was high as time was running out to complete all my clinical requirements to graduate. After a particularly stressful day in the clinic, I left early with a bad migraine. They were all bad, but this one was particularly awful. A classmate drove me back to my apartment, and I remember calling my family to let them know (just in case I died). My mother and sister drove down to stay with me that night.

At the time, I did not have any medication prescribed for migraines. Since they only occurred occasionally, I had not seen a doctor for migraine treatment. I would usually take some over-the-counter pain medicine and try to sleep it off. But no amount of Tylenol or Advil was going to touch this headache. I had a prescription pain medication left over from having wisdom teeth extracted, so I took one. I took one of these pills every 4–6 hours as prescribed. It only mildly blunted the pain and made me sleepy. I felt nauseous. I remember dragging myself to the door to let my mother and sister in before crawling back on the couch. During the next few hours, I experienced stroke-like symptoms. My speech was slurred, and my mouth drew to one side. My poor mother and sister could not understand what I was saying, but they did their best to make me comfortable. The headache seemed to last forever. I had never been to the emergency room with a migraine before, but this probably should have been one of those times. Fortunately, the headache finally passed, and I was able to get some sleep that night with my mother and sister watching over me.

Clinic awaited the next day, and I had to pass a patient requirement in order to graduate (no pressure). I made it through the day and completed my clinical requirement. I am not sure how I made it because I was not functioning at normal capacity. Since hygiene school was incredibly stressful, I had several more (thankfully, less severe) migraines during that time, but they came more frequently. After graduation, the headaches were less frequent and less severe. That is when I learned firsthand what stress can do to you. It usually was, and still can be, a trigger for me.

Fortunately, I have not experienced stroke-like symptoms to that extreme since then. But the neurological symptoms are still there. I now notice tingling, involuntary muscle contractions in my arms and legs, slurred speech, lack of mental clarity, dizziness and, of course, the visual changes. A few have sent me to the emergency room. After college, I saw a neurologist who confirmed that I have classic migraines (migraine with aura). I tried the migraine-specific drugs called triptans (sumatriptan and naratriptan) but with little to no relief and some side effects I did not enjoy. I was also treated for anxiety, which probably helped. Later, I was referred to a doctor specializing in complementary and alternative medicine for another condition (fibromyalgia). He suggested some supplements, stress reduction and gentle exercises such as yoga and tai chi. The supplements made me feel better and worked better for migraines than the prescription medicine I had tried. They were also much cheaper and had no unpleasant side effects. I began using 5-HTP for prevention and treatment of migraines. The other supplement contained magnesium, which I would later learn could help with migraines and fibromyalgia. (We will discuss non-drug treatment options in chapter 8).

After about a month of incorporating his recommendations into my routine, I felt less pain and my headaches improved as well. I still had the occasional migraine, but I noticed the pain was less intense and they did not seem to last as long.

Over the course of the next several years, I slacked off my supplements and exercise routine, and ended up having a migraine. Most were milder than what they were before. Usually, I would take a 5-HTP and find relief, but occasionally, they were so bad that nothing seemed to help. A few times they were bad enough to send me to the emergency room.

The triggers for these migraines varied. Sometimes I could pinpoint the cause. Stress seemed to be a big trigger for me. Occasionally I blamed it on hormone changes, but this was not the norm. Certain perfumes or cologne would trigger one, so I learned to stay away from the perfume counters in department stores and avoid candle shops. I try to keep a good distance between me and someone wearing cologne or perfume (especially certain scents or if it is overpowering). I even had a migraine after going down the detergent aisle at the grocery store. Now I just hold my breath or let my husband pick up the detergent. I also try to avoid cigarette smoke.

Bright lights, especially flashing lights, are known triggers for me as well. I try to avoid flickering fluorescent lights, or any flashing light, because they have triggered a migraine on more than one occasion. The flickering of a computer screen can also become a problem if I spend too much time at one. Loud noises have always bothered me, but they normally do not trigger a migraine unless accompanied by something else such as flashing lights.

Allowing my blood sugar to drop can provoke a migraine. After waiting too long to eat lunch one day, I learned the hard way not to do that again. I had gone past the point of feeling hungry and that was enough to trigger a migraine. Now I have a regular meal schedule with snacks as needed. This helps with all headaches, not just migraines.

Staying hydrated helps me avoid all types of headaches as well. After working outside in the yard one hot summer day, I learned what dehydration can do. While gardening in the hot sun with the temperature approaching 90, the sweat was running into my eyes and my shirt was wet. I kept telling myself that I would go in to cool off and get some water as soon as I finished what I was doing. Unfortunately, I had waited too long. Shortly after going inside and drinking some water, an aura started letting me know a migraine headache was on the way. Now I take breaks and drink plenty of water as needed based on the temperature, how much I am sweating and as I feel thirsty. Drinking water all day long even while working at my desk helps keep headaches less frequent. Water or flavored water (without artificial sweeteners) is my preferred drink for staying hydrated.

Some food additives can trigger a migraine for some people. One day while working in a dental office, I learned aspartame was not my friend. I never drank diet drinks but this day, I tried one with lunch (because that was the only option . . . well, besides water). I found that to be a bad idea. Now I avoid anything with aspartame. I also avoid caffeine. This helps me avoid the temptation to drink something just for the caffeine. For me, caffeine does not seem to be a trigger for migraines, but it provokes heart palpitations and is not good for someone with anxiety issues. It is possible that monosodium glutamate (MSG) and some other food additives bother me, but I cannot prove that they are triggers for me, at least not by themselves. But I typically avoid foods that I know contain added MSG.

Over the years, I began noticing some food triggers. Chocolate tasted good, but I did not like the headache that followed. After eating a sandwich with fresh homegrown tomatoes, I developed a migraine. I tried tomatoes and tomato sauce again two more times with same results, so sadly tomatoes are no longer in my diet. Citrus fruits seemed to bother me, so they became off limits. This is where a diet diary helps. I took a food tolerance test (Pinnertest) and found that I reacted to five foods including egg yolks, cocoa, onions, barley, and arugula.

This food reaction or intolerance is not the same as an actual food allergy such as to peanuts or shrimp where a person develops an anaphylactic reaction that causes swelling of the throat, trouble breathing, etc. A food allergy is an immediate reaction and requires medical attention.

I was not surprised by cocoa since I knew chocolate was an issue, but the others surprised me. However, none of these other foods by themselves had ever triggered a migraine for me. And tomatoes, the one food I knew for sure triggered a migraine, did not show up on the test as being an issue. Citrus fruits did not show up as an issue either.

So, my advice is to use a diet diary to see what tends to trigger your migraines. There is some controversy on the accuracy of food allergy tests, and they can be quite expensive. And just because you may have an intolerance to a certain food does not mean they trigger migraines. Foods can affect you in other ways. A diet diary and migraine log are your best resources when it comes to determining food triggers for you. We will discuss food triggers and how to do an elimination diet for migraines in chapter 6.

Sleeping too much or too little has also prompted one. After sleeping late one morning and getting way more than my usual eight hours, I developed a migraine soon after getting up. Having a regular sleep schedule really helps with all types of headaches. After waking up with a migraine a few mornings, I started looking at sleep as a trigger. Tracking my sleep (using a fitness tracker) and trying to improve the quality of my sleep has made a big difference in how I feel overall. Having a comfortable mattress and pillow also makes a difference in sleep quality. I have tried multiples of both over the years and found that it does impact how I feel in the morning. Currently, I have an adjustable Sleep Number® bed and use a water pillow purchased from Amazon. Getting adequate support for my neck and back has made a comfortable difference in my sleep.

Changes in weather or even seasons of the year can trigger a migraine as well. A thunderstorm seemed to appear out of nowhere one summer day, which caused a sudden change in barometric pressure. That was enough to trigger a migraine for me and has made me more conscious of weather patterns. Unfortunately, we have no control over the weather, but I can make sure I avoid any other triggers that may make a migraine more likely. Changes in the seasons still tend to provoke a migraine for me, likely due to seasonal allergies. These days, I typically experience one or two migraines a year, and they tend to coincide with the change of season in spring and fall. Fall is my worst time followed by spring. I have gone a whole year without a migraine, but I usually still have one a year (typically in the fall). Minimizing exposure to allergens does seem to help.

It was not until last year that I had a migraine that came close to the one I experienced in college. I was working at the local health department. It was a typical day at work, and it seemed to hit me out of the blue. It started with the aura. I was in the middle of a session with a client, but fortunately I had a colleague with me who could take over while I excused myself to treat a migraine. Unfortunately, the 5-HTP (which is the only thing I had with me since I had not had a migraine in a long time) did not help. It progressed into a terrible headache accompanied by neurological symptoms. I could not control my legs and arms, and my hand became contracted. Nausea and vomiting eventually set in. It is the first time I ever passed out with a migraine. It is a little embarrassing when they call the medical team for you as you are lying half-conscious in the hallway. A coworker had to drive me to the ER. It took hours to get the pain under control and for my vision to return to normal. As often happens, a CT scan was ordered to rule out a stroke or tumor. I have had so many CT scans over the years; I feel like my brain should glow. Even though I knew it was a migraine, the ER doctors must rule out worst-case scenarios. I understand their protocol, but it is annoying that treatment, including pain medication, is held until after the scan results come back. As usual, the scan came back normal. After receiving IV fluids and multiple medications, I was released about four hours later. My husband drove me home where I slept on the couch for the rest of the evening. I had received so much medication in the ER and was so exhausted from the migraine that I did little more than sleep for the next two days. I received prescriptions from the ER including Naproxen and Tramadol for pain and ondansetron (Zofran) for nausea which my husband picked up for me.

As a word of warning from my personal experience, I had been taking amitriptyline for the past six months for another issue (GI-related) but was bothered by the side effects. Even though I was taking a small dose and had been tapering off, evidently coming off the medication was a stressor on my body. I believe that was a factor in triggering this migraine. So, if you are on a medication, especially medications that help regulate neurotransmitters like antidepressants (SSRIs, SNRIs, MAOIs), be cautious if you stop taking them. Talk to your healthcare provider for tips on how to safely come off any medication. It may save you some pain and suffering.

I slowly returned to normal and went back to work the following week. I followed up with my primary care doctor and described the episode I experienced. Since I had not seen a neurologist in years, I was referred to one for further evaluation. A magnetic resonance image (MRI) was ordered and the results were just as I suspected: completely normal. This is why migraines are so difficult to diagnose. All test results come back normal because migraines do not show up on x-rays. Imaging only helps to rule out other causes of headache. Due to my known history of migraines, the provider gave me samples of diclofenac potassium powder (Cambia®) in case I had another one. I had one migraine after that visit (likely triggered by allergies due to the change in season—hello, spring). The Cambia® helped. I was thankful to have something at home that I could take instead of going to the emergency room, especially since this occurred during the COVID-19 pandemic, and I really did not want to go to a hospital during this time.

I have noticed a few changes in my migraine symptoms as I have grown older. The pain is usually less severe than when I was a teenager or in my early twenties. The neurological symptoms, however, seem a little worse. As I approach menopause, I expect some changes in my migraines to occur, and I expect them to stop eventually. We will see.

I know everyone experiences these headaches differently, but I hope sharing my story gives you some insight into yours and lets you know that you are not suffering through this alone. For females, the good news is migraines typically diminish or completely disappear after menopause due to decreased fluctuations in estrogen. I know this is not true for everyone, but for most of us, it is something to look forward to.

There is no cure for migraine, but with some knowledge and development of a few coping skills, you can improve your migraines. For some, there are other causes of migraines not listed here. If you suffer from migraines as a secondary headache, seek help for treatment of that condition first.

Everyone is unique, but I believe that by avoiding certain known triggers and using some treatment options presented in chapters 7 and 8, you can lessen the impact of migraine and improve your quality of life. If sharing my experience and knowledge from over 30 years of migraines can help you or someone you love, then I hope you are blessed by this book and share it with fellow migraineurs.

SECTION 2

Prevention and Treatment of Migraine

— 5 —
Prevention of Migraines

NOW THAT WE better understand what happens inside our brain during a migraine and some common triggers for migraine, we will focus on how to avoid triggers that may set off the chain of events leading to a migraine. As with most diseases, prevention is far better than treatment, and that holds true for migraine.

Triggers vary from person to person and may change over time. Some triggers may be more likely to cause a migraine for you than for others and one trigger by itself may not always be enough to provoke a migraine. There may be a dose-dependent response to triggers. In other words, being exposed to a small amount of a trigger (like a food or scent) may not be enough to cause a migraine; however, if you are exposed to a trigger in a larger quantity or multiple triggers together, then the likelihood of a migraine is increased. As we discuss potential triggers and how to avoid them, you may start noticing which ones affect you.

Addressing Triggers to Avoid Migraine

Dietary-Related

Dehydration

Staying hydrated—consuming enough water or fluids to support the physiological functions of your body—is important. This can help prevent other headaches as well. Many of us are mildly dehydrated from lack of fluid intake on any given day. Being in a hot climate, sweating, running a fever or taking certain medications can make this worse. The amount of water needed depends on your age, body size, activity level, climate, health status and even the calories you consume. For example, if you have a fever, live in a hot climate or exercise at a high intensity, you will need more. The more calories you consume (especially from dry foods such as grains, meats, nuts and seeds), the more fluid your body needs to process those calories.

Due to this variation in need for water, the Food and Nutrition Board (FNB) of the Institute of Medicine does not give a Dietary Reference Intake (DRI) for water. Instead, they list an Adequate Intake (AI) amount based on available data. The AI for total water intake listed for healthy men (ages 19–50) is 3.7 Liters per day. That equals 125 ounces, or 15.5 cups. For healthy women (ages 19–50), the AI is 2.7 Liters per day (91 ounces), or 11.5 cups. Fluid requirements decrease slightly in the over 50 age group but not much. Research studies showed that about 80% of fluid needs are met through beverages and 20% from foods such as fruits and vegetables[1] (think berries, cucumbers, lettuce, and watermelon).

To estimate your individual fluid needs, take your weight in pounds and divide by two. This easy rule of thumb takes in consideration your total body mass rather than your age and gender. This gives you a rough estimate of how many ounces of fluid you should consume daily. You can adjust from there as needed.

For example: A 150 lb. female would need 75 ounces of fluid per day (150 ÷ 2 = 75). That equals about four (20-ounce) bottles. If you prefer to think of it in cups, we can do a little math. Since there are 8 ounces in one cup of fluid, we divide 75 by 8 to get 9.4 cups. That means a 150 lb. female should drink roughly 9 and a half cups of fluid daily.

Our result in this example is two cups less than the AI determined by the FNB. But 9.5 cups would equal about 80% of the recommended fluid intake considered adequate. Remember that the other 20% comes from foods like fruits and vegetables. Acquiring your daily fluid needs is best achieved by drinking clean, filtered water and eating several servings of fruits and vegetables every day.

Despite the controversy surrounding the contribution of caffeinated, sugar-sweetened, or alcoholic beverages to daily fluid requirements, it appears there is insufficient evidence to state that caffeine, sugar, or alcohol causes water loss in significant enough amounts to impact hydration. Therefore, these beverages do count toward your daily fluid intake according to the FNB. However, it is best to include water as part of your daily fluid to prevent overconsumption of caffeine, sugar, or alcohol, which may lead to excess weight gain or dependency. Coffee and tea act as mild diuretics, so you will not get the full benefit of hydration from these beverages. Allow your body to be your guide in staying hydrated. If you feel thirsty, have a dry mouth or your urine is a dark yellow, then drink more water.

Food Triggers

Food as a sole cause of migraine is believed to be uncommon. However, most people with migraines report at least one known food trigger. As mentioned in chapter 4, chocolate and tomatoes are a trigger for me. To determine if certain foods may be triggering a migraine for you, I recommend keeping a food and headache log. If you are having frequent headaches, this will be the best way to determine if there is a link between a food and your migraines.

Food allergy testing can provide insight into which foods may cause a reaction for you, but they do not specifically test for migraine triggers.

Just because you do not tolerate a certain food well does not mean that it causes a migraine. That food may cause inflammation or other symptoms instead. Testing can be expensive, and the accuracy is controversial. I was tested for food intolerances because I had the opportunity to try it for free. The results provided me with information to investigate further but did not specify which foods I should avoid for preventing migraines. If you have the money, being tested is fine. Just do not expect it to tell you everything you need to know. Trial and error and elimination diets are still the gold standard in detecting food intolerances. Once you have a diet diary and headache log, working with a doctor or a registered dietitian with experience in working with people with migraine may help you find the answers you need. We will explore more about the dietary component in migraine in chapter 6.

Changes in Blood Sugar

The amount of sugar (glucose) in our blood fluctuates all the time whether we have diabetes or not. Your body attempts to regulate blood glucose levels within a healthy range (usually between 70 and 140 mg/dL). Some conditions such as hypoglycemia (low blood sugar) or diabetes can interfere with normal blood sugar balance.

Lifestyle factors influence blood sugar fluctuations as well. Skipping meals is one of the most common causes of a drop in blood glucose. Going too long between meals (typically meaning more than 5 or 6 hours) can cause you to feel tired, weak, and shaky. It may lead to a headache for most people. But for people that are prone to migraines, it may trigger an attack. The brain does not function well without adequate glucose, so your body has a way of letting you know that you need to eat. Having a regular meal schedule helps you avoid blood sugar fluctuations.

Listening to your body is important. If you start feeling hungry, you should eat. Waiting too long can cause that dip in blood glucose that will make you feel bad. I recommend eating about every 4–5 hours throughout the day. Include a variety of food groups to make sure you get adequate complex carbohydrates, lean protein, and healthy fats. Avoid eating too much at any one meal. Eating smaller meals makes you more likely to be hungry at the next mealtime and reduces the burden on your digestive system. If you get hungry between meals, try adding a small snack, but avoid loading up on sugar. The high sugar intake may boost your energy level temporarily, but the inevitable crash or drop in blood sugar level later may make you feel worse. Fasting or extreme diets can also lead to a drop in blood sugar. Following an extremely low carbohydrate diet can trigger a headache in most people. If you are prone to migraines, avoiding these extremes in your diet can save you a lot of misery.

Lifestyle Related

Sleep

We all need sleep, but for some a good night's rest can be elusive. If you are not getting adequate sleep (6–8 hours per night) or you are not achieving a good quality sleep, you may notice more migraines. Sleep can directly or indirectly impact headaches. When we do not get enough sleep, our body does not get the restorative time at night it needs to heal. We may find ourselves more agitated, anxious, fatigued or not thinking clearly. Lack of sleep is a risk factor for several medical conditions.

To get adequate sleep, try improving your sleep routine. This will help you properly wind down at the end of the day and prepare yourself for sleep. This includes turning off electronics or other things that may overstimulate your brain. Dimming the lights can help increase melatonin production, which promotes sleep. Avoiding exercise before bedtime allows your body time to relax. Avoid eating a heavy meal or large snack within 2–3 hours before bedtime. Your food should be fully digested prior to trying to sleep. Lying down after a big meal also increases your risk of acid reflux, which can interfere with sleep. Alternatively, if you are hungry, try eating a small snack before bed. If you are preoccupied with feeling hungry, it will be harder for you to drift off to sleep. Remember to allow time to digest.

Also helpful for a healthy sleep routine is having a set bedtime. People with a regular sleep schedule find it easier to get into the rhythm of sleep and may naturally feel sleepy once their body is used to going to bed at a certain time. Get up around the same time each morning. Sleeping in may be tempting, but if you sleep much longer than usual, you may find headaches are more likely. Also, you can never make up for lost sleep during the week by sleeping longer on weekends. Allow your body the rest it needs by allowing enough time each night for sleep.

Find ways to relax prior to bedtime. Taking a hot bath or listening to soothing music can prepare you for sleep. If reading makes you sleepy, try reading a book you enjoy. Make sure it is nothing that will upset you or keep your interest too long so that it prevents you from going to sleep. Try some relaxation or deep breathing techniques before bed. Guided imagery can help clear your mind if you are having trouble falling asleep. Progressive relaxation can help release tension in your body. If you are still struggling to sleep, try aromatherapy using lavender. You can diffuse the oil or mist on your clothes or bedding.

Make sure your bedroom is comfortable. Preferably you want a cool (not too cold), quiet, dark room. Adjust your temperature and use an automatic thermostat, if possible, to keep you comfortable all night. If there are outside noises bothering you that you have no control over, try wearing ear plugs or using ambient noise to drown it out. Use blackout curtains or shades to block outside light. Remove all sources of light in the room including cell phones or other items with lights while you sleep. You want to distance yourself from the distractions as much as possible.

If you are still having problems sleeping, ask your healthcare provider if supplements may be helpful. I like magnesium, melatonin, 5-HTP, and L-theanine. If none of these tips improve your sleep, speak to a sleep specialist. Once your sleep quality improves, you will notice waking up feeling refreshed and ready to tackle the day.

Stress

Stress is probably the most common cause for migraine. Whether it is physical, mental, or emotional stress, the impact on our bodies is undeniable. While a little stress can be a good thing, chronic stress can cause a host of issues. A brain under stress is more likely to provoke a migraine attack. The stress response sparks a cascade of chemical reactions involving neurotransmitters that may lead to a migraine. More on the role of neurotransmitters in the development of migraines can be found in chapter 8. The tension your body stores when stressed may also lead to migraines. If you are clenching or grinding your teeth, clenching your fists, tightening your neck or shoulders, or having TMJ issues, practicing relaxation techniques can be helpful.

Being stressed makes sleep more difficult, which can lead to sleep deprivation, also a known trigger for migraine. Stress can also cause an upset stomach. It was believed long ago that there was a connection between the gut and migraines since vomiting often led to relief. The gut-brain connection in migraine may involve neurotransmitters since serotonin can affect the gut and cause nausea.

There may be times when you notice a migraine after a stressful event is over. This is the letdown phase following acute stress, which can lead to a migraine. Additionally, physical stress such as intense exercise or sex may also trigger a migraine for some people. Learning to cope with stress can go a long way in preventing a migraine attack. Here I will describe a few techniques or methods that can make a difference.

Mindfulness – This means living in the moment, being aware of what is going on around you and how you feel. Practicing mindfulness allows you to be a spectator. You may feel anxious, worried or even depressed. Stop and allow yourself to feel those feelings without judgment or trying to change it. This can help you discover what makes you feel a certain way and may help with anxiety. By observing how your body feels without panicking, you can focus on your breathing and relaxation techniques to alleviate symptoms. Just take some deep breaths and focus on something pleasant until your body starts to feel calmer. With some practice, you can assess your body, thoughts and feelings and respond to them in a calm way.

Meditation – This is like mindfulness, but your focus is taken off yourself and how you feel and placed onto something else. You can focus on a picture, a candle or repeat a saying over and over. This helps you clear your mind and only focus on one thing. It takes some practice but over time it can help you feel more relaxed. By practicing meditation (or prayer, a form of meditation) on a regular basis, you will feel more comfortable with it and it will become easier to deal with stress.

Biofeedback – This technique teaches you how to use your mind to control some subconscious reactions in your body. It is similar to but more intensive than mindfulness and meditation. Biofeedback uses sensors to measure heartrate, blood pressure, respirations, skin temperature and muscle activity. It gives you a visual indication of how your body responds to stress and to stress reduction techniques. By seeing how your body responds to these techniques, you can design a routine for stress reduction that works for you.

Yoga – This Eastern tradition of combining focused breathing and meditation with body movement is effective for reducing stress and calming the nervous system. When certain relaxing poses are used, yoga can be extremely helpful in stretching tight muscles and releasing tension. The emphasis on taking deep full breaths helps increase the oxygen supply to the brain. Deep breathing alone is a simple and free natural headache remedy. Taking a yoga class can be beneficial to get you started. There are also some good videos available for free on YouTube. I do not recommend hot yoga or difficult poses as they may trigger migraine.

Tai Chi – This ancient Chinese practice is a relaxing exercise that uses slow movements to calm the mind and body. Tai chi has proven effects on mood, fatigue, and sleep. I personally found tai chi to be helpful and surprisingly calming. There are videos available to help you get started if classes are not offered near you. It is easy on the body and does not require special equipment or skills. You can practice in your living room or outside for some fresh air.

Exercise – Exercise in general is good for the body. It does not have to be strenuous or last for hours to be effective. Start by taking a walk. If you cannot go outside due to weather, a treadmill works fine too. Try listening to relaxing music or upbeat music for some motivation, depending on your mood. Walking outside gives you the added benefit of experiencing nature. Being surrounded by nature and the energy that comes from the earth can be therapeutic. Enjoy the birds singing, water flowing, gentle breezes and the beauty nature brings for added benefits.

Massage – If muscle tension seems to plague you, try massage therapy. A good therapeutic massage can get the blood flowing. This is important because blood carries nutrients that help nourish all tissues of the body. It can help relax muscles and release your body's natural pain killers known as endorphins. Getting a massage, even a short massage, on a regular basis may help alleviate the tension that can lead to tension-type headaches and may also be beneficial for migraines. You can utilize massage at home by rubbing your neck and shoulders, massaging your temples, your feet or any other area that feels tense.

Counseling – Sometimes we find ourselves stuck in thought patterns that create stress in our lives. A certified counselor trained in cognitive behavioral therapy can help identify those negative thoughts that contribute to our stress level. Changing these unhealthy thought patterns may lessen the tension we hold in our body. If there are things in your past that caused great pain, this can help you deal with those. Allowing negative feelings to build over time can lead to chronic health problems, and medication will not get rid of those thoughts or feelings. Dealing with any feelings or frustrations you have can improve your outlook on life. You may still have migraines, but hopefully they will become less frequent and/or less intense in time.

Environmental Triggers

In chapter 3, we discussed some possible triggers you may encounter that are best avoided. Sometimes they are impossible to avoid. If you find yourself in a situation where you may be exposed to some of these triggers, it is okay to remove yourself from the environment. You do not owe anyone an explanation. If you choose to explain your triggers and migraine, that is totally up to you. Not everyone will understand, but someone who cares about your well-being will sympathize once you tell them how migraines affect you and why you choose to avoid those things that may trigger one.

Scents

Some possible triggers you may come across in the environment include scents of any kind such as those found in perfumes, colognes, candles, fragrances in soap and cleaning products. The smell of gasoline, paint or cigarette smoke can be a trigger. Not every smell may be a trigger for you, but through experience you will likely find what smells you need to stay away from. This may be an allergic response that activates histamine. Using nasal sprays or antihistamines may help.

Changes in Season

For some people, a change in season may precipitate migraines. As certain allergens become more prominent (especially in the spring and fall), they may trigger a histamine reaction for some. Histamine can cause inflammation and provoke a host of chemical changes in the body. If you notice more migraines at a specific time of year, you may be sensitive to some things in your environment. Antihistamines or certain nasal sprays that block mast cells from producing histamine might help.

Weather

Another factor which we have no control over is weather. Sudden changes in barometric pressure, such as during a thunderstorm, can bring on a migraine. If you know weather is changing or sense a storm coming, try some of the preventive techniques to help prevent or at least lessen the attack provoked by changing weather.

Light and Sound

Bright or flashing lights and loud noises may be a trigger for some people. This is thought to be due to overstimulation of the brain, which may trigger neuron activity that excites the brain. The excitability of the neurons then may provoke changes in blood vessels causing aura and/or pain in people prone to migraine. It is believed that people with migraines are more sensitive to these external stimuli. Even the flickering light from computer screens or other electronic devices may be too much for a migraineur, especially when exposed for prolonged periods of time. In theory, calming the nervous system may help alleviate the episode associated with sensory stimulation. If you can avoid bright or flashing lights and extremely loud noises, that may be your best bet.

———

Although not necessarily related to triggers discussed in this chapter, I want to mention two other therapies here that some may find beneficial. Chiropractic care and acupuncture or acupressure can help alleviate pain. If cervical issues seem to be a trigger for migraine for you, a chiropractic adjustment may help. This can be a safer alternative to other more invasive treatments for neck and back pain. The ancient Chinese medicine practice of acupuncture involves inserting needles along key meridians and has been used for migraine prevention; acupressure works in a similar way. Studies have been conducted regarding the benefits of acupuncture in migraines with some good results.

People rarely have a sole factor for migraines. There is usually a build-up of factors which lead to a migraine. Those factors may include anything we have discussed in this chapter and may depend on the amount of that trigger to which we are exposed. Learning to identify your migraine triggers will go a long way toward prevention.

Since there are multiple components in food that can trigger a migraine, we will take a detailed look at food and how to identify dietary triggers in chapter 6. If avoiding these triggers still does not improve migraine for you, we will discuss preventive treatments in chapters 7 and 8, including drugs and non-drug therapy. It is important to work with a qualified healthcare provider to help you navigate through the many options and find what is safe and works best for you.

— 6 —
Diet and Migraine Headaches

ACCORDING TO THE Association of Migraine Disorders, about 25% of migraine sufferers report having food triggers for migraine.[1] It is believed that food as a sole cause of migraine is uncommon, but many people experience significant relief with dietary changes. If you suffer from frequent migraine headaches, an elimination diet would be advised. For some people, food can provoke a response in the body that triggers a migraine. To be considered a migraine trigger, a food must cause migraine-related symptoms within 24 hours of the time it is consumed, and must do so more than half the time that the food is eaten.[2] In this chapter, we will explore the possible dietary triggers for migraine and ways to discover if food is a trigger for you.

Determining which foods might be a trigger for your migraine can be complicated. Not everyone will have the same triggers. It can also depend on the amount consumed. Foods do not always trigger a migraine immediately. Adding to the difficulty, a food may trigger a migraine at one time but not another depending on other factors. It can also change over time. If you have frequent migraines but are not sure if food is a factor, I recommend starting with the most common food triggers first. Be careful when eliminating certain foods or food groups from the diet. Unnecessary avoidance of foods can lead to nutritional deficiency and place social and financial burdens on you and your family. You will need to replace foods eliminated with equally nutritious foods to avoid nutrient deficiencies, so I recommend working with a registered dietitian to help you navigate the nutritional implications of doing an elimination diet. A registered dietitian can help you determine which foods to exclude and how to reintroduce them back into your diet. To find a registered dietitian in your area, go to the Academy of Nutrition and Dietetics website at www.eatright.org and use their "Find an Expert" listing. Ask if they work with people with migraines when you contact them to make sure you are getting someone qualified to help you.

The number of food triggers for migraine in an individual is generally small. There is rarely a need to eliminate multiple foods or entire food groups from the diet. About one-third of people with frequent migraines will experience a significant reduction in headache frequency on an elimination diet and a small percentage (less than 10%) will become headache free.[3]

Common Food and Beverage Triggers for Migraine	
Aged Cheese	Beer
Chocolate	Coffee
Citrus fruits	Milk
Corn	Tea
Cured Meats	Wine (especially red)
Fish and Shellfish	
Garlic and Onion	
Legumes (peanuts, pinto beans, soybeans, black-eyed peas)	
Nuts	
Pork	
Tomato	
Wheat	

One study reported the frequency with which specific foods triggered migraine in migraine-prone individuals during a food challenge test.[4] Based on the percentage of times a food triggered a migraine in this study, frequency of these foods as triggers are listed in order from most often to least often.

Milk (43%)

Chocolate (29%)

Hot dog (14%)

Cheese (14%)

Fish (10%)

Wine (9%)

Coffee (9%)

Garlic (5%)

Eggs (5%)

How Foods Can Trigger Migraine

Substances in foods that modify vascular tone or foods that promote hypoglycemia (low blood sugar) are thought to be the mechanisms by which food can trigger migraine. Components of food that can affect blood vessels include tyramine, phenylalanine, phenolic flavonoids, alcohol, food additives (aspartame, sodium nitrate, MSG) and caffeine.[5] If you are accustomed to drinking caffeine-containing beverages, withdrawal from caffeine can precipitate vascular or tension headaches but does not directly cause migraines. In some cases, caffeine can relieve migraines, possibly due to its vasoconstrictive effects on blood vessels in the scalp. Chronic daily headaches can be caused by excessive use of caffeine (more than 1200 mg, or 5–6 cups of coffee per day).[6]

Foods may trigger migraine by provoking an immune response from an allergic reaction or a physiological response to chemicals in foods. Some foods are more likely to cause this reaction than others. Milk, fish, and eggs are common food allergens that may promote inflammation. Chocolate, cheese, and wine contain *biogenic amines*. Biogenic amines are nitrogen-containing compounds synthesized usually from amino acids (building blocks of protein) through the action of enzymes or microbes during metabolism. For example, histamine is a biogenic amine derived from the amino acid histidine. These nitrogen-containing compounds mimic the actions of the sympathetic nervous system (the system responsible for the fight-or-flight response). Biogenic amines include histamine, tyramine, octopamine and phenylethylamine. Histamine is released from mast cells in response to allergic reactions or tissue damage. Due to the close proximity of mast cells to blood vessels and the effects of histamine on blood vessels, we see the potential for histamine reactions promoting migraines by the influence on blood flow to the brain.[7] Caffeine is a biogenic amine called methylxanthine that is commonly found in coffee, tea and soda. Nitrites found in processed meats such as hot dogs also affect blood vessels. Exposure to enough of any of these foods or substances could trigger a response in those prone to migraines.

Unfortunately, due to the complexity of effects food can have on the brain and blood vessels, there is no single lab test that will indicate which foods and additives are responsible. Allergy tests usually rely on detecting immunoglobulins, also known as antibodies, produced in response to exposure to certain substances. The usual allergy tests are not helpful in determining which foods to eliminate from the diet to prevent migraines. This is because the hypersensitive reaction that skin testing is designed to detect (which is Immunoglobulin E- or IgE-mediated hypersensitivity) is not an important or frequent cause of migraine in adults. Researchers suggest that immune response associated with foods in migraine sufferers are of the Immunoglobulin G (IgG) type. In most cases, a food-specific IgG is a normal response to foods commonly consumed, and therefore, the benefit of IgG in the diagnosis of adverse reactions to foods is controversial. If an IgE-mediated hypersensitivity is a cause of migraines, other signs of allergy are also evident, almost without exception.[8] These may include symptoms of the respiratory tract, skin, or digestive tract.

Categories of Foods as Potential Migraine Trigger

It is time to examine food components implicated in more detail and explain ways these foods may contribute to migraine. We can divide these food components into six categories. The categories are alcohol, food allergies, biogenic amines, nitrates and nitrites, food additives, and other pharmacologically active chemicals.

Alcohol

Beer, wine and other alcoholic beverages contain biogenic amines and sulfites. These are more likely to trigger a migraine than the alcohol itself.

Food Allergies

A food allergy is a condition in which a certain food triggers an abnormal immune response. This abnormal response is caused by the immune system mistakenly recognizing some proteins in food as harmful. In response to this, the body launches protective measures, including the release of histamine, which causes inflammation. True food allergies can be divided into IgE or non-IgE antibody responses. The top ten foods most commonly implicated in food allergy reactions are cow's milk and milk products, eggs, peanuts, tree nuts, fish, shellfish, corn, soy, seeds and wheat. Symptoms of a reaction to these foods can occur anywhere from a few minutes to a few hours after exposure, and may include swelling of the face, mouth or tongue, difficulty breathing, itchy rash, hives, diarrhea or vomiting. In extreme cases, it can lead to anaphylaxis, a life-threatening emergency.

Food intolerances can cause some of the same symptoms and be mistaken for food allergies. However, a food intolerance does not involve the immune system and is not life-threatening. An example is lactose intolerance in which the lactose in milk is not sufficiently digested due to a lack of the enzyme lactase. This results in lactose passing into the colon where bacteria ferment it, resulting in the production of gas that leads to gastrointestinal symptoms such as abdominal pain, flatulence, bloating and diarrhea. Food intolerances can produce annoying symptoms, but they do not damage the gastrointestinal tract and are not dangerous.

Because food allergies can trigger the release of histamine, this may explain the correlation between food allergens and migraine headaches. Food allergies must be identified first as these are the most serious. Any true food allergen should be avoided. Doing so can help reduce histamine release and may improve headaches for some people. An allergy test measuring IgE would be appropriate to identify food allergies. Removing food allergens from your diet may or may not provide relief from migraines. There are other food components that may be involved that do not necessarily include a food allergy.

Biogenic amines

These nitrogen-containing compounds found in foods may contribute to migraine by affecting blood vessels, either by narrowing (vasoconstriction) or widening (vasodilation). The biogenic amines most frequently implicated in triggering migraine headaches are histamine, tyramine, octopamine, phenylethylamine and putrescine.[9]

Sources of *histamine* in the diet include fish, certain vegetables, fermented foods and beverages, and cured meats.

Sources of Histamine in the Diet				
Chocolate	Strawberry	Cheese	Bologna	Beer
Egg white	Eggplant	Sauerkraut	Pepperoni	Wine
Fish	Tomato	Soy sauce	Salami	Ale
Shellfish	Spinach			Lager

Sources of *tyramine* in the diet include some fruits, aged cheese, fermented foods, vinegar, and foods containing vinegar.

Sources of Tyramine in the Diet		
Avocado	Sauerkraut	Vinegar
Banana	Sour cream	Mustard
Broad bean (fava) pods	Smoked salmon	Pickles
Aged cheese	Pickled herring	Relish
Chicken liver	Yeast extract	Salad dressing
Sausage	Peanuts	Wine

Sources of *phenylethylamine* in the diet include chocolate, aged cheese, and red wine.

Sources of Phenylethylamine in the Diet
Chocolate
Aged cheese
Red wine

Some foods contain multiple biogenic amines which may increase their effect on blood vessels making them more likely to provoke a migraine. Limiting the amount of these foods consumed at one time may help.

Nitrates and Nitrites

The mechanism by which nitrates and nitrites may trigger migraine is not completely understood. There appears to be two effects involved and may differ depending on the individual. If a headache arises immediately upon consuming nitrate-rich foods, it may be connected to vasodilation caused by the release of nitric oxide (NO). Another cause may be the release of calcitonin gene-related peptide (CGRP) or glutamate.[10] Nitrates and nitrites are used in foods as preservatives and coloring agents. Some foods containing nitrates or nitrites include cured meats (hot dogs, salami, bologna, pepperoni, luncheon meats, ham and bacon), smoked meats and fish (smoked bacon, smoked salmon), and aged cheeses.

Food Additives

Some food additives commonly associated with migraine include artificial colors (especially azo dyes such as tartrazine) and preservatives (like sulfites and benzoates) that act as histamine-releasing agents. Monosodium glutamate (MSG) as well as some herbs and spices (like cinnamon, cayenne, curry spices, nutmeg and thyme) are also associated with histamine release. This may be due to the presence of natural benzoates. Artificial sweeteners, especially aspartame, may also be a problem. Aspartame is a combination of two amino acids (L-aspartic acid and L-phenylalanine). It is 180 times sweeter than sugar. It is found in diet soda, sugar-free gum and many diet products as well as some medications and supplements.

Other Pharmacologically Active Chemicals

Food is not the only source of these components implicated in triggering migraine. Other chemicals that may have a drug-like effect include caffeine, theobromine, theophylline and aminophylline. These can affect the blood vessels surrounding the brain as well as other smooth muscles in the body. These chemicals, referred to as *methylxanthines*, can be found in foods and beverages such as coffee, tea, cola drinks, cocoa and chocolate (except white chocolate). But they can also be found in nonprescription supplements such as caffeine tablets and weight loss aids (diet pills).

Identifying Food Triggers

Keeping a record of foods eaten and headache symptoms can help you detect possible food triggers. The record should be kept long enough to include at least three migraine episodes. This may take several weeks if episodes are infrequent. You may reveal specific food trigger(s) if the reaction is immediate due to food allergy. However, this is not a common finding. You may also notice a dose-related response to food intolerance triggers such as histamine, tyramine, or food additives. This can occur if a food substance builds up over time and exceeds your tolerance threshold.

An elimination diet followed by a food challenge remains the gold standard for detecting food triggers in migraine. If a food is reintroduced, after being eliminated for at least two weeks, and a migraine occurs within 24 hours, on more than one occasion, it should be eliminated from the diet. It can always be reintroduced again later to see if the food remains a trigger for you.

There are several different ways to conduct an elimination diet. You may choose to remove the foods that you suspect trigger a migraine first. This is known as a *selective elimination diet*. If you are not sure which, if any, foods are triggering a migraine, you may choose to eliminate the most common food culprits. These would include the foods and beverages listed in the table of *Common Food and Beverage Triggers for Migraine.* Food additives or naturally occurring chemicals you may choose to avoid include artificial colors, benzoates, MSG and sulfites. Although less common, these additives have been reported as food triggers in migraineurs, but evidence is inconclusive as to these being the actual cause. Paying attention to the ingredient list on food packages can help you detect common dietary culprits. It may be difficult to determine the specific trigger, but over time you can narrow down the lists of suspects. This will make it easier to use an elimination diet to discover foods you may need to avoid.

In some extreme cases, you may need to follow a *few foods elimination diet*. This diet allows only a few "safe" foods in the diet. Due to the restrictive nature and increased risk of nutrient deficiencies, this diet should not be followed more than 7–10 days. These very restrictive diets are not recommended in young children (under the age of 13) or for pregnant or lactating women. You should always work with a registered dietitian while following an extreme diet to guarantee you are getting adequate calories and nutrients, so you can avoid deficiencies which may lead to health problems later. Because a very restrictive diet should be followed only under the supervision of a qualified professional, a few foods diet will not be covered in this book.

Conducting an Elimination Diet

My recommendation is to start by eliminating suspected trigger foods first. If you are still experiencing frequent migraines, then try eliminating the common food culprits. The most frequently suspected triggers of migraines and other types of headaches are the *biogenic amines*, especially histamine and tyramine, so trying a time-limited biogenic amine-restricted diet may yield the results you need. This can help eliminate the need for a more restricted diet.

Once you have determined which elimination diet you should follow, prepare yourself both physically and mentally for the challenge. A drastic change of diet will go much easier if you plan ahead. Before beginning, follow the steps listed below. As always, consult a registered dietitian if you need help getting started.

1. Make a list of foods to include in your diet. It is much easier to focus on what you *can* eat rather than on what you cannot. Any foods that are not suspected triggers or not listed in the common trigger foods or beverages are fair game.

2. Plan meals and snacks ahead of time. This is where a menu can come in handy. Make an outline of your meals and snacks for an entire week or an entire month. This takes the guessing out of "what's for dinner?" and saves you time when grocery shopping.

3. Go shopping. Stock up on plenty of "safe" foods to guarantee you have options and are not tempted to grab a food that is off-limits. Make sure you have plenty of choices for meals and snacks that are easy to prepare or take with you. Cooking at home can simplify things because dining out makes it much harder to control or even know which foods and additives restaurants use.

4. Keep track of foods and headaches. Writing down when you ate, what you ate, how much you ate and where you ate provides important

details when looking for food triggers. Keeping a log of headaches, not just migraines, can help you identify a link to certain foods over time. Record when the headache started and how long it lasted. Jot down any other symptoms you experience as well, such as aura or other neurological issues. For women, you may also want to note times of menstrual cycle to see if that may be the correlation instead of food.

5. Remember that this diet is only temporary. You will begin reintroducing foods back into your diet once the elimination phase is over. It is not necessary for you to eliminate these foods from your diet forever. You will only avoid those foods that prove to trigger a migraine for you.

Once you are prepared, you will follow the elimination period for four weeks (or longer if needed) to include at least three or four episodes of migraine. This allows enough time to get suspected foods out of your system. It also gives you time to see whether you feel better once you remove these foods. Just keep in mind that you may feel worse on days 2–4 of the elimination diet. Consider this the withdrawal period. By days 5–7, you should feel better and see significant improvement by days 7–10. If all triggers have been removed from the diet, your symptoms will disappear by the third week.[11] If you have any skin or gastrointestinal issues, these will usually improve as well, if they are diet related.

Record your meals and snacks during this period and log any symptoms you experience. If symptoms remain after the four-week elimination period, then migraines may be related to food triggers or allergens remaining in the diet or your symptoms are unrelated to food. Keep a separate log and jot down any other factors such as stress level, sleep changes, exercise, exposure to environmental triggers or change in routine. You will want to try eliminating other causative factors for best results. Once other triggers are removed, extend the elimination diet for another two weeks. If the diet contains sufficient nutrients from other foods, there is no risk from extending the elimination diet. This helps to differentiate food as a trigger versus other causes.

While following the elimination diet, food should be washed and cooked with distilled or filtered water if possible. Unfiltered water may contain contaminants that could cause reactions. Avoid cooking in pots or pans with nonstick coatings as the coating may react with foods cooked in them. Glass is the preferred non-reactive container for cooking, but iron skillets are also okay.

Be sure to eliminate all dietary components that may cause a reaction. This means avoiding breath mints, chewing gum, coffee, tea (including herbal) and diet drinks. Try to avoid other factors such as mouthwash, tobacco products (including cigarettes) and unnecessary over-the-counter medications. Continue all necessary prescription medicines as prescribed by your healthcare provider. If you suspect a prescribed medication may be contributing to your symptoms, talk to you doctor for advice on other options or how to stop a medication safely. Some medications should never be stopped abruptly as there can be serious consequences.

Food Challenge Phase

At the end of four weeks (or more if needed), you will begin to slowly reintroduce the eliminated foods one at a time. Since it is hard giving up your favorite foods, I recommend adding these back first. You will add one food (or food component) to the foods you have been consuming. Include that food or food component in your diet several times a day over four days or until you have a reaction to it. This gradual introduction and accumulation of a food over four days allows enough time to reveal both an immediate-type reaction and a delayed response.

Always start with the purest form of a food first, and then work up to combination food components. For example, for dairy, start with milk and then try ice cream or cheese. If you love a combination food like pizza, you will add each component of pizza back one at a time. This will include cheese, tomato sauce, meat such as pepperoni or sausage, and pizza crust. You can choose to add these back in any order you prefer. It will take four days of testing for each ingredient. Determining the guilty food can possibly allow you to still enjoy pizza if you omit the offending culprit. This food challenge phase will take longer than the elimination phase. Keep in mind that you may find you react to a certain food more strongly after eliminating it from your diet for several weeks. This may reveal a hidden food allergy that you may not have noticed when you were eating it frequently. For dose-dependent trigger foods, such as biogenic amines, you may not notice a reaction until the third or fourth day after you have accumulated enough of it in your diet.

At the end of the four days of each food trial or challenge, assuming you have added enough of it into your diet, you should know if that food is a problem for you. If you have no reaction to eating the food daily for four days, then you can consider that food as safe and continue to enjoy it as you add the next foods back. For foods that cause a reaction, you may choose to add that to your "foods to avoid" list and remove it from your diet. If you really love a trigger food, you may choose to include it, perhaps in smaller amounts, aware that it may have consequences. This is your choice, but now you know so that you can make an informed decision.

Repeat the food challenge process with each food until you have added all the foods you want to include back to your diet. If one food alone is not enough to trigger a migraine attack, see if combinations of foods are an issue. If so, this means that the accumulation of certain food components has exceeded your tolerance threshold.

If food is an issue, you may find that you feel better overall and maybe you will discover certain foods that cause other issues for you aside from migraine as you go through an elimination phase. Keeping a diet and symptom log along with noting other non-food triggers is important to make sure you gain the most insight out of the process. It takes time, but the payoff is improved quality of life and fewer migraines.

— 7 —
Pharmaceutical Treatment of Migraine

AFTER IDENTIFYING AND eliminating all known triggers, you still get a migraine. Now what? Life happens and we cannot control everything. Knowing what to do whenever a migraine hits is just as important as trying to prevent one. In this chapter, we will discuss treatment options for migraine attacks. Whether you have occasional or chronic migraines, getting proper treatment is important. Allowing the pain to perpetuate does not help your physical or psychological well-being and can lead to a vicious cycle of pain. Fortunately, there are more options today than we had just five years ago. As research continues, hopefully we will have more options available. In this chapter, we will explore pharmaceutical options currently available for the treatment of a migraine attack as well as preventive treatments for chronic migraine management.

It is believed there are many contributing factors to migraine, so it makes sense that one medication may work for some but not for everyone. Finding what works for you can be a game of trial and error. Working with a caring, compassionate health professional can get you help quicker. If one medication is not working, let your healthcare provider know so they can try something else. Always discuss any concerns you may have with them. Some medications may not be recommended for you due to your medical history or family history. Also, some medications can interact with others, so your doctor or pharmacist can discuss the risks and determine what is best for you. Even if you are taking over-the-counter medications to treat a migraine, you may want to consult a specialist to see if there are better options, especially if you are not getting the results you desire.

Medications

There are two primary forms of medications used in migraine treatment: acute and preventive. Acute medications are used to treat a migraine attack by relieving pain and helping to stop the migraine from progressing. Preventive medications are used if migraines are chronic (occurring at least eight days per month) to help reduce the frequency or at least shorten the duration of migraines.

Acute Medications

There are three classes of migraine medications primarily used to treat a migraine attack. These include prescription and over-the-counter medications. While other supportive medications may be given to alleviate symptoms such as nausea during a migraine, we will focus on the main three used in acute migraine treatment.

Analgesics

These pain relievers include acetaminophen (Tylenol®), and a class of drugs known as non-steroidal anti-inflammatories (NSAIDs) like ibuprofen (Advil®, Motrin®) and diclofenac potassium (Cambia®). These are available either over the counter or as a prescription. Some will include caffeine due to its vasoconstrictive properties, which may help them work better. Another option includes opioids like hydrocodone (Vicodin®). These drugs use an opioid combined with another pain-relieving drug such as acetaminophen.

These medications do not treat the cause of migraine but help reduce inflammation and lessen the associated pain to make the patient more comfortable until migraine runs its course. These are most effective for mild to moderate migraine pain. It is not recommended to use this type of medication often as they can lead to rebound headaches and increase the risk of chronic migraines. Opioids can be addictive and should only be used if other treatments are not working.

Triptans

This class of drugs known as selective serotonin (5HT1) agonists were the first migraine-specific medication available. Sumatriptan (Imitrex®) was patented by GlaxoSmithKline and became available in 1991.[1] Other variations (zolmitriptan, naratriptan, eletriptan, frovatriptan, rizatriptan, almotriptan) with various brand names became available soon after. These are available by prescription only and come as tablets or dissolving tablets, nasal sprays, or injections.

Triptans target two specific receptors on sensory nerves and work by affecting blood vessels and serotonin levels. If the pain of migraine is caused by dilation of blood vessels, the action of vasoconstriction may help improve pain. Consequently, they can also constrict other blood vessels and are contraindicated in people with heart disease, high blood pressure or at risk of stroke. This is the first class of drugs designed exclusively for treatment of migraine, and they are considered the gold standard for acute migraine treatment.

Ergotamines

Although not widely used now, this was the first class of drug used to treat migraine starting in the 1950s. Ergotamine, like triptans, work by affecting blood vessels causing vasoconstriction. Drugs in this class usually contain caffeine (Cafergot®). Since ergotamine is not as targeted as triptans, they are typically less effective and have more risks. These are usually reserved for severe migraine or for those not responding to other treatments. This medication class is not advised for people with heart disease or high blood pressure due to the vasoconstrictive action, which can increase the risk of a heart attack or stroke.

Drugs used for acute migraine treatment should not be used more than ten days per month. Using them more frequently can cause rebound headaches and can progress into chronic migraines.

Preventive Medications

If you experience migraines more than four days per month or they are very disabling, you may need to consider preventive therapy. These medications or treatments are used in addition to medication for treating attacks. This can help lessen the frequency and intensity of migraine and reduce your need for acute treatment. These options may help prevent development of chronic migraine. There are a few different types of drugs used for migraine prevention. These include medications used to treat high blood pressure, seizure disorder, and depression. They can help with chronic migraines due to the actions they exert either on blood vessels or on neurotransmitters in the brain.

Antihypertensives

The four classes of medications used to treat high blood pressure include beta blockers, calcium channel blockers, angiotensin receptor blockers (ARBs) and angiotensin converting enzyme (ACE) inhibitors. They work to lower blood pressure by different actions in the body and may be helpful for people with migraines. This can be especially true if blood pressure tends to be elevated, which can be a factor provoking headaches. Each class of medication is listed and described below.

Beta Blockers – Beta blockers work by blocking the effects of the hormone epinephrine, also known as adrenaline. This causes your heart to beat more slowly and with less force, which lowers blood pressure. Beta blockers have drug names that end in "-lol" such as atenolol, propranolol or metoprolol. While these can be effective for some people, they are not ideal for those that already have a slow heartbeat or low blood pressure.

Calcium Channel Blockers – Calcium Channel blockers work by inhibiting the entry of calcium ions into the smooth muscle of the blood vessels and myocardium. This relaxes the smooth muscle decreasing peripheral vascular resistance and dilates coronary arteries causing a decrease in blood pressure. These drug names end in "-pine" such as amlodipine and nifedipine. While helpful in lowering blood pressure, these are not recommended for those with low or normal blood pressure.

Angiotensin Receptor Blockers (ARBs) – ARBs work by blocking the receptor of a hormone called angiotensin II. By blocking the receptor for this hormone, it prevents angiotensin from increasing blood pressure through vasoconstriction and promotion of water retention. Drug names in this class will end in "-sartan" such as losartan or valsartan. As with most drugs, these are contraindicated during pregnancy and lactation. These may interfere with other medications or certain health conditions, so speak to your doctor if you have any concerns.

Angiotensin Converting Enzyme Inhibitors (ACE Inhibitors) – Similar to ARBs, ACE inhibitors block angiotensin II, but they work by inhibiting the angiotensin converting enzyme. This interferes with the conversion of angiotensin I to angiotensin II, thereby preventing the action of angiotensin II on blood vessels. These drug names end in "-pril" such as lisinopril, enalapril, and monopril.

As with all drugs, there are possible side effects. Your doctor may need to monitor you more closely if you are taking any of these medications. Discuss the pros and cons of these medications with your healthcare provider to see if the benefit outweighs the risk. If you experience side effects and are considering stopping these medications, do so only with the advice of your doctor. Stopping some medications abruptly can have serious consequences.

Anticonvulsants

Anti-seizure medications can be used in the prevention of migraine. These medications such as topiramate (Topamax®), valproic acid (Depakote®) and gabapentin (Neurontin®) work by calming neurons in the brain. Since migraines are thought to be related to hyperactivity in the brain, this can help reduce the frequency and/or intensity. These can be helpful as a preventive drug for chronic migraine. Discuss possible side effects of these drugs with your healthcare provider to see if the benefit outweighs the risks. Always consult your doctor before making any changes to your medication dose or routine.

Antidepressants

These medications work on neurotransmitters in the brain that seem to be involved in migraine. Amitriptyline (Elavil®) and venlafaxine (Effexor®) are antidepressants that have been around for years and have commonly been used in prevention of migraine. Both work on serotonin and norepinephrine, but venlafaxine also works on dopamine to inhibit reuptake of these neurotransmitters in the brain. Side effects are possible, so talk to your doctor about any concerns you may have. These medications should never be stopped abruptly. If you need to stop an antidepressant medication for any reason, consult your doctor for how to come off the drug safely. Be sure to tell your healthcare provider all other medications and supplements you are taking to avoid any potential interactions.

Next Generation Migraine Medications

There are some gene-specific therapies that have come on the market recently. They target a specific protein or peptide which may help reduce pain and whole-body effects of migraine. Researchers discovered that calcitonin gene-related peptide (CGRP), a protein that is released around the brain, is involved in migraine. They believed if we could stop CGRP, we could stop a migraine. As a result, several pharmaceutical companies went to work on a way to stop CGRP and developed monoclonal antibodies against CGRP and the receptor to which CGRP binds. During a migraine, levels of CGRP greatly increase and are found in pain fibers surrounding the blood vessels around the brain, meninges and trigeminal nerve. This triggers expansion of blood vessels, inflammation and the cascade of pain and other familiar symptoms of migraine. By blocking CGRP activity, the pain signal is not initiated. This new generation of medications may offer hope to migraine sufferers who have not found relief from other therapies. We will discuss the available options of this next generation migraine medication below.

CGRP Inhibitors

These new drugs target CGRP by either blocking the peptide itself or the receptor it acts upon. CGRP medications can be divided into two distinct groups: the larger sized group (called *monoclonal antibodies*) and the small-sized compounds (referred to as *gepants*). We will discuss both types.

Monoclonal antibodies (mAb) are large molecule CGRP-blocking drugs requiring injection because they cannot cross through the blood-brain barrier into the brain. They are designed to prevent migraines and are usually given monthly via self-administered subcutaneous injection. The first FDA-approved drug of this kind appeared on the market May 2018. The drug erenumab (Aimovig®) was soon followed by other drugs in this class, fremanezumab (Ajoy®) and galcanezumab (Emgality®). According to Dr. Stewart Tepper, the director of the Dartmouth Headache Center and professor of neurology at the Geisel School of Medicine, research studies show minimal side effects in study participants. The most common side effect was pain at injection site. However, the potential problems of blocking CGRP on a long-term basis, if any, are not yet known. Caution is advised during pregnancy or in those with high blood pressure. While promising, these mAb medications are no miracle drug. However, they have been shown to decrease the frequency of migraine in many patients by at least 50%.[2]

More recently, another type of drug that blocks CGRP came on the market. These new, smaller molecules can cross the barrier into the blood around the brain and can be taken orally as tablets or dissolving tablets. These medications, referred to as *gepants*, have been studied mostly for the acute management of migraine attacks and can be taken as needed. These medications work by blocking CGRP receptors, thereby blocking pain transmission to the brain along the trigeminal nerve and blood vessels surrounding it. Drugs in this category first gained FDA-approval in December 2019 and include ubrogepant (Ubrelvy®) and rimegepant (Nurtec®). These drugs should be taken at the first sign of migraine.

Ditans

Another new migraine-specific medication appeared on the market in February 2020. This latest addition to the migraine arsenal, lasmiditan (Reyvow®), is the first FDA-approved oral serotonin 5-HT1F receptor agonist. It is indicated for use in acute migraine treatment. It works similarly to triptans but targets a more specific receptor (5-HT1F) to block signals along the trigeminal nerve without affecting blood vessels. It may be a good option for those experiencing side effects from or that do not respond to triptans. Since lasmiditan does not cause vasoconstriction, it may be safer for those with a history of cardiovascular disease. The limitation of lasmiditan is that it is a controlled substance and has the potential for causing sedation. Due to its recent appearance on the market, it has not been time-tested as other medications have, so caution is advised.

Other Medication Options

Another treatment option for those who have not responded to any of the previous medications listed may be onabotulinumtoxinA, known by the brand name Botox®. This option is FDA-approved for migraine prevention only in people experiencing 15 or more migraines per month. It is administered by injection into head and neck muscles every three months and works to prevent activation of pain receptors in the brain by blocking the release of chemicals involved in pain transmission. Due to the potential side effects, this should be considered as a last resort. It is also an expensive option that may not be covered by all insurance carriers.

How to Know if Your Migraine Medication is Working

According to Dr. Rebecca Michael, an assistant professor in the department of neurology at the University of California, San Francisco, medications used for acute migraine attacks should provide relief or a return to function within two hours after taking the medication. How well you respond to a medication within 24 hours after taking it should also be considered. If the migraine comes back or you have significant pain again in four to six hours after taking it, that is a sign your acute medication might not be working as well as it should. If you have been on a treatment plan for at least two months, discuss any of these observations with your healthcare provider so they can determine whether to continue this medication or try a new treatment plan.

If you experience a migraine once a month or once every few months, then medication to treat acute attacks should be sufficient; however, if you experience more than four migraines a month or find them disabling, you should be on both a preventive and an acute medication, according to Dr. Michael. Working closely with a headache specialist is the best way to come up with a treatment plan for migraine management that works for you. To find a headache specialist in your area, check out additional resources listed in the back of this book.

Fortunately, there are a few more options available on the market for treating or reducing migraine frequency and intensity, but preventing a migraine is better by far. As researchers learn more about the brain and what happens during a migraine attack, we can be better equipped with prevention strategies. But based on what we know about migraines so far, we can make informed decisions on what will work best for us individually. In chapter 3, we discussed triggers for migraine. We know that changes in the brain provoked by sensory neurons causing blood vessel changes or chemical imbalances have been implicated in triggering migraines. With those in mind, next we will look at some ways to support our brain to lessen the effect these changes have on us.

— 8 —
Natural and Non-Pharmaceutical Treatment for Migraine

ADDRESSING DIET AND lifestyle factors first is always the best option. You can often get good results without side effects. Based on the factors currently believed to be involved in migraine development, we will discuss natural ways to influence those in this section.

The Serotonin Factor

Various factors can alter the nervous system and possibly contribute to an attack. One factor implicated in migraine is the major neurotransmitter serotonin, also known as 5-Hydroxytryptamine or 5-HT for short. Research has shown that migraineurs tend to have low levels of serotonin in their brain. This is how antidepressants such as amitriptyline can work to prevent or reduce frequency of migraine attacks. They increase serotonin signaling in the brain to help compensate for the low level. This is believed to be how they treat depression as well. Targeting serotonin also led to the development of the classes of drugs known as triptans and more recently ditans.

These medications have been helpful in treating a migraine attack; but unfortunately, they are not useful for prevention and come with a list of potential side effects. The good news is there are ways to boost your serotonin level without pharmaceutical drugs.[1]

One natural way to boost serotonin levels is exposure to bright light like sunshine or light therapy. This can lift our mood and make us feel better. Regular exercise can have the same effect. A healthy diet includes good quality proteins such as eggs, cheese, nuts, salmon, and turkey, which help increase production of serotonin. Meditation helps to relieve stress and minimizing stress can help boost serotonin levels as well. Sometimes there are factors we cannot control, and diet and lifestyle may not be enough. In this case, supplementation with a good quality nutritional supplement can be beneficial. We will discuss some supplements here for general education.

5-HTP and L-tryptophan

To naturally boost serotonin (5-HT) levels in our brain, we need to be able to produce it from 5-Hydroxytryptophan (5-HTP). 5-HTP is only found in food in small amounts but it is a chemical involved in the metabolism of tryptophan to serotonin. Tryptophan is an essential amino acid present in several foods including oats, bananas, dried prunes, milk, tuna, cheese, bread, chicken, turkey, peanuts, and chocolate. To convert tryptophan into 5-HTP, the presence of folic acid, vitamin B6, magnesium, calcium and iron are required along with a specific enzyme. Once 5-HTP is produced, vitamin B6, magnesium, zinc and vitamin C are required to convert it into serotonin (5-HT). If your diet is low in tryptophan or any of the other nutrients required for conversion, then supplementation may be needed. The production of 5-HTP is the rate-limiting step in serotonin synthesis. This means if 5-HTP production is impaired, serotonin cannot be produced.

Tryptophan ▶ **5-HTP** ▶ **Serotonin**

Supplements can help provide the necessary components for serotonin production. L-tryptophan is an amino acid available in supplement form, and 2–4 grams of L-tryptophan taken daily has been shown to be as effective at preventing migraine attacks as the ergot-derived prescription drug methysergide.[2] Another supplement option is 5-HTP, which has been used for several diseases where serotonin is believed to play an important role. Taking 5-HTP provides the direct precursor for serotonin production without the conversion from tryptophan. The supplement can be taken before bed as it may cause drowsiness. These supplements typically come in 50 or 100 mg doses. I always recommend starting with the lowest dose and gradually increasing to monitor for tolerance. Since 5-HTP can increase serotonin levels, it should not be taken along with other medications or supplements that affect serotonin production. Too much serotonin can lead to serotonin syndrome, a potentially life-threatening condition.

Melatonin

A natural compound our body produces to help us sleep is melatonin. While serotonin production is boosted by exposure to light, melatonin production is triggered by darkness. As the sun goes down, melatonin production is signaled to prepare us for sleep. It is often found in lower than normal levels among migraine sufferers (especially during an attack) and may play an important role in migraine pathology. Since melatonin is produced in the pineal gland, some researchers hypothesize that migraines are triggered by an irregularity in pineal gland function. By correcting this imbalance with melatonin supplementation, some patients experience improvement in symptoms.[3] Melatonin may help in other ways as well. It has been shown to possess potent antioxidant and analgesic properties. Interestingly, melatonin is made from serotonin. Therefore, if serotonin levels are low, melatonin production is impaired. Melatonin taken in supplement form at a dose of 3 mg daily over 12 weeks was shown to be effective in reducing migraine attacks by 51%.[4] Melatonin has been found to be safe with few side effects. Start with a low dose and gradually increase until sleep is achieved. Improvements in the amount and quality of sleep may be beneficial in migraine prevention.

Tryptophan ▶ **5-HTP** ▶ **Serotonin** ▶ **Melatonin**

SAMe (S-adenosylmethionine)

SAMe is a naturally occurring substance produced by the body involved in a variety of important biochemical processes, especially involving the central nervous system (CNS). It is also available as a nutritional supplement derived from the amino acid methionine and the nucleic acid adenosine triphosphate. It can increase serotonin and some studies suggest long-term supplementation with SAMe may relieve pain for migraine sufferers.[5]

The Nutrient Factor

Certain nutrients are critical for proper brain function. If one nutrient is lacking, this can have a cascade effect on the entire brain chemistry. Since there are critical nutrients involved in regulating these biochemical processes, vitamins and minerals could play a vital role in migraine prevention. Nutritional supplements may especially be helpful for people who have a nutrient deficiency. We will discuss the nutrients most researched and recommended to lessen the frequency and intensity of migraine. Most of these can safely be taken along with other medications, but as always, consult your healthcare provider before taking to make sure they are safe for you.

Magnesium

A deficiency of magnesium has been associated with depression, interference with the release of neurotransmitters (like serotonin), the aggregation of platelets, and constriction of blood vessels. All these processes are believed to be involved in migraine. Magnesium may play a role in stabilizing neural excitability and vascular tone, which can help with migraine prevention. One pilot study evaluated forty people with migraine and found that during a migraine attack, 50% of them had low levels of magnesium in the brain. The intravenous (IV) administration of magnesium appeared to reduce the pain of the migraine in about 50% of these patients.[6] For women, low levels of magnesium were more commonly found during menstrual migraine compared to migraine occurring at other times. Magnesium deficiency may play a role in menstrual migraines.

Magnesium is widely found in foods including green leafy vegetables, nuts, seeds, legumes, whole grains, bananas, avocados and dark chocolate. Pumpkin seeds are an excellent source. The Recommended Dietary Allowance (RDA) for magnesium as set by the Food and Nutrition Board (FNB) ranges from 310 to 420 mg for adults, based on age and gender.[7] Some people may not get enough magnesium from their diet or may not absorb magnesium due to a lack of stomach acid, perhaps from long-term use of acid-blockers. In these cases, magnesium supplementation may be beneficial. Several small studies have found that oral supplementation of magnesium may reduce the frequency and severity of migraine attacks. In one study from 1996 of 81 people with migraine who were randomly assigned magnesium or a placebo, magnesium supplementation reduced the frequency of attacks by 41.6% compared to 15.8% in the placebo group.[8] More recently, a 2008 study compared magnesium supplementation given to thirty patients compared to ten patients given placebo. The study found that treatment with magnesium resulted in a significant decrease in frequency and severity of migraine attacks.[9]

While it is possible to test blood magnesium levels, it may not be useful to do so. Only a small percentage (1%) of magnesium is found in the blood. The remainder is found in tissues such as bone and muscle. Even in cases of magnesium deficiency, the blood magnesium level remains normal although total body stores are depleted. Other conditions that may contribute to a low blood magnesium test include diabetic acidosis, chronic kidney disease and hemodialysis, chronic pancreatitis, chronic alcoholism, malabsorption issues, pregnancy, or excessive loss of body fluids.[10]

Magnesium does not occur alone; it is usually bound to another salt or protein. There are several different forms of magnesium to choose from and some are better absorbed than others. I generally recommend magnesium glycinate, magnesium citrate, or magnesium L-threonate. Other forms available include magnesium oxide and magnesium malate. Magnesium oxide is not as readily absorbed and has a greater potential for causing stomach upset or diarrhea. However, it is one of the least expensive forms of magnesium supplements and has been used in research studies.

Magnesium supplements come in many forms including powder, capsule, liquid and tablets. Topical magnesium is available as a cream or ointment, but there is controversy regarding the amount that is absorbed through the skin. Soaking in an Epsom salt (magnesium sulfate) bath is another way to add magnesium. Since magnesium supplementation is generally safe, I recommend a good quality, bioavailable (easily absorbed) magnesium supplement and start with a small dose. You can gradually increase the amount as needed to achieve the desired effect. Diarrhea is the most common side effect from magnesium supplementation. If this occurs, cut back on the dose or stop the magnesium for a while.

There are some conditions for which magnesium supplementation may not be advised such as kidney disease. There are also some drug interactions possible with magnesium supplements. Talk to your doctor before starting a magnesium supplement to make sure it is safe for you. The Tolerable Upper Intake Level (UL) for supplemental magnesium is 350 mg. However, according to the American Migraine Foundation, daily doses of 400 to 500 mg of magnesium may help prevent migraines in some people. This may be especially effective for migraines related to menstruation, and those accompanied by visual changes or aura. A dose of 600 mg daily was used in some studies showing effectiveness for migraine prevention. The dose needed varies by individual and may be best tolerated taken in smaller, divided doses throughout the day. Magnesium should be consumed with calcium in a ratio of 1:2. Calcium supplementation should not be taken without magnesium. Increasing magnesium from food and/or supplements may help some migraine sufferers, but it may take a while to see improvement, so do not expect immediate results.

B Vitamins

The B vitamins known as riboflavin (B2), folate (B9), pyridoxine (B6) and cobalamin (B12) may all play a role in control of migraines. Some researchers propose that low mitochondrial energy reserves can cause migraine and some B vitamins play a role in mitochondrial function. An increase in homocysteine levels can trigger migraine attacks. Researchers have found evidence that homocysteine (an amino acid occurring in the body as an intermediate in the metabolism of methionine and cysteine) is involved in triggering migraine. Vitamin B6, B12 and folate are required for homocysteine catalyzation. Adequate amounts of these vitamins may decrease the severity of migraine with aura, making these vitamins potentially useful as preventive agents.[11]

Riboflavin (vitamin B2)

Riboflavin has been rated as having moderate to strong evidence for migraine prevention. Riboflavin serves several roles in the body, including the maintenance of mitochondrial function. Because some types of migraines are thought to occur due to mitochondria not working properly, it is believed that riboflavin may be helpful in people suffering from metabolic-related migraines.[12]Foods high in riboflavin include milk, yogurt, liver, beef, eggs, poultry, seafood, almonds, brown rice, dark green leafy vegetables such as spinach, and fortified grain cereals or oatmeal. Common riboflavin doses for migraine sufferers are 400 mg daily over a period of about three months. For migraines, a riboflavin supplement alone rather than taken along with other B vitamins seems to work best, so be sure to get a riboflavin supplement and not a vitamin B complex. There are few side effects noted at that dosage level, although you may have bright yellow urine and rarely diarrhea can occur. Pregnant women should always discuss taking any kind of vitamin supplementation with their physicians. Excess riboflavin may cause skin issues such as itching, numbness or burning sensations. If you are suffering from unbearable migraine attacks, it may be worth talking with a healthcare provider to see if riboflavin would be a good fit for you. Unlike most medications, riboflavin is very affordable and safe.

Folate (vitamin B9)

A folate deficiency may be due to lack of folate or folic acid in the diet. It may also be caused by a missing enzyme due to a genetic defect which leads to the inability to convert folic acid to the active form folate. A blood test can easily detect a deficiency of folate. If a genetic defect is suspected, supplementation with the appropriate form of folate is needed. A lack of folate is associated with elevated levels of homocysteine, which may play a role in migraine with aura. Food sources high in folate include liver, spinach, asparagus and Brussels sprouts. The U.S. Food and Drug Administration (FDA) has required folic acid to be added to certain grain products since 1998 to help prevent deficiencies. The RDA for folate is 400 micrograms (mcg) for adults and goes up to 600 mcg during pregnancy.[13]

Pyridoxine (vitamin B6)

A deficiency of vitamin B6 may be correlated with migraine in multiple ways. Along with folate and vitamin B12, low vitamin B6 is implicated in high levels of homocysteine. As discussed earlier, vitamin B6 is also required for the conversion of 5-HTP to serotonin. The RDA for vitamin B6, according to the FNB, is 1.2 to 2.0 mg per day for adults depending on gender and whether pregnant or lactating. Food sources rich in vitamin B6 include fish, beef liver and other organ meats, potatoes, some fruits and fortified cereals. The UL established by the FNB for vitamin B6 is 100 mg. Supplementation with vitamin B6 along with folate and vitamin B12 may be beneficial in migraine, but work with a qualified healthcare provider to help navigate the intricacies of dosing and possible contraindications. Excess doses of any nutrient have the potential for harm.

Cobalamin (vitamin B12)

A deficiency of vitamin B12 can occur due to a lack of vitamin B12 in the diet (more likely in vegans) or due to pernicious anemia (condition where the person is unable to absorb B12). Good food sources of vitamin B12 include animal products: fish, meat, poultry, eggs, milk and milk products. Vitamin B12 is generally not present in plant foods, but fortified breakfast cereals can be a good source for vegetarians. The RDA for vitamin B12 is set at 2.4 to 2.8 mcg for adults. No UL has been set for B12 due to the relative safety of vitamin B12 from food or supplements.

Supplemental vitamin B12 is available in liquid, tablets, sublingual lozenges or by intramuscular injection by a doctor. Low levels of vitamin B12 are implicated in high homocysteine levels. When present in sufficient quantities along with vitamin B6 and folate, B12 may help lower homocysteine levels, making it useful for migraine prevention.

Vitamin E

Vitamin E has many roles including antioxidant, inhibition of platelet aggregation (blood clotting), anti-inflammatory and immune enhancement.[14] It is believed the role it plays in the anti-inflammatory process may explain the beneficial role of vitamin E for menstrual migraines. A true deficiency of vitamin E is rare but possible in those following a low-fat diet. Food sources of vitamin E include nuts, seeds, vegetable oils, green leafy vegetables and fortified cereals. The RDA for vitamin E is 15 mg daily for adults. If your dietary intake is adequate, supplementation may not be recommended. In high doses, vitamin E may interfere with blood clotting and interact with certain medications.

Vitamin C

Vitamin C, also known as ascorbic acid, is a water-soluble vitamin required for collagen production, protein metabolism and production of certain neurotransmitters. It also functions as an antioxidant in the body and has been shown to regenerate other antioxidants within the body, including vitamin E.[15] Vitamin C has been studied in treating neurogenic inflammation in migraine patients through its antioxidant properties.

Good food sources for vitamin C include fruits (especially citrus fruits, kiwi, strawberries) and vegetables (tomatoes, potatoes, red and green peppers, broccoli and Brussels sprouts). Vitamin C is destroyed by heat during cooking and with prolonged storage. It is water-soluble and can leach out if submersed in water such as while boiling. Consuming fruits and vegetables in raw form is best.

The RDA for vitamin C ranges 75–90 mg in adults with higher amounts needed during pregnancy or lactation. Smoking depletes vitamin C, so higher intakes are recommended for smokers. A deficiency of vitamin C can lead to scurvy. In higher doses, vitamin C has low toxicity and is not believed to cause serious adverse effects. The most common complaints are diarrhea, nausea or abdominal cramps. However, due to possible interactions with certain medications, consult a healthcare professional for advice on supplementation.

Coenzyme Q10 (CoQ10)

Coenzyme Q10 is naturally produced by the body and is found inside the body's muscle cells, especially in the heart muscle. It is key to the functioning of the mitochondria, the powerhouse inside cells that produces the energy the cell needs. CoQ10 has antioxidant properties and can reduce damage to cells. It is available as a dietary supplement, but is also found in several foods including beef, chicken, salmon, boiled eggs, broccoli, spinach, oranges, roasted peanuts and canola, olive and soybean oils. CoQ10 is fat-soluble and best absorbed when taken with a meal. Our body makes less of it as we age, and some medications (particularly statin drugs) can lower CoQ10 in the body.

CoQ10 is considered an antioxidant vitamin and has been rated as having moderate evidence for migraine prevention by the American Academy of Neurology and the European Federation of Headache Societies. This may be due to the role it plays in mitochondrial function and its possible anti-inflammatory effect. CoQ10 may be particularly effective in pediatric migraine.[16]

Studies have shown evidence that CoQ10 supplements may help prevent migraines. One study found that among 31 patients who took 150 mg of CoQ10 daily for three months, 61% of them reported at least a 50% reduction in the number of days they had migraine attacks. No side effects were noticed among study participants. Another small study of 42 migraine sufferers compared CoQ10 (taken as 100 mg three times daily) to an inactive placebo. In that study, the supplement was three times more likely than placebo to reduce the number of migraine attacks.[17] Side effects noted, included stomach upset and skin rash. Other possible side effects of CoQ10 supplementation include nausea, vomiting, diarrhea, heartburn, loss of appetite, abdominal pain or discomfort, tachycardia (rapid heartbeat) and a mild increase in liver enzymes.

CoQ10 may interact with other medications or supplements. Consult your doctor before taking CoQ10 if you are taking a blood pressure medication, blood thinner, cholesterol medicine or a tricyclic antidepressant. Your doctor may want to monitor blood glucose since CoQ10 can lower blood sugar. Avoid if pregnant, planning to become pregnant or lactating.

Herbal Supplements

In addition to the vitamins and minerals we discussed, there are some herbal supplements that are used for natural migraine prevention. There are several natural migraine therapies featured in the 2016 Recommended Treatments for Complementary Therapies issued by the American Academy of Neurology (AAN) and the American Headache Society (AHS). We will look at two with the most evidence for migraine prevention.

Butterbur

One herb with strong evidence for migraine prevention is butterbur. It contains chemicals that may help relieve swelling and reduce inflammation, both thought to be associated with migraines. Although controversial in the past due to concerns with pyrrolizidine alkaloids (PA) contamination, which can cause liver damage, certain brands labeled "PA-free" are now considered safe. Researchers used a butterbur extract standardized to 15% petasin and isopetasin (the active ingredients in butterbur), which was free of the liver-damaging PAs. Using a specific extract from the butterbur root over 16 weeks can reduce the number, severity and duration of migraine headaches. Butterbur extract was shown to reduce the number of migraine headaches by almost half. Doses of at least 75 mg twice daily appear to be necessary for best results.[18]

Feverfew

Another herb with moderate evidence for migraine prevention is feverfew. It is a flower in the daisy family that has been used for decades to help relieve migraines. It is available in liquid, tea and capsule form. It can be taken daily or at the first sign of an attack. A few small studies have shown a reduction in frequency of migraines when taken daily. Feverfew is not considered harmful but can thin the blood, so do not take it if you are pregnant or take blood thinners. Some potentially serious side effects include allergic reactions, mouth ulcers, anxiety or upset stomach. Avoid feverfew if you are allergic to ragweed. In some cases, it can actually cause headaches.[19]

Always discuss supplements with your healthcare provider to avoid supplement-drug interactions and potential side effects.

The Hormone Factor

It is believed that hormones, particularly estrogen, play a role in migraine. This seems obvious because women are three times more likely to experience migraine than men. It also seems obvious since migraines are more prevalent at certain ages where female hormones fluctuate more and are influenced by hormone-based pills like birth control. It has been estimated that more than 40% of women in America have had to deal with a migraine at one time or another. This discrepancy in occurrence seems to be contributed to a drop in estrogen that occurs either right before or after menstruation.[20] This can vary among individuals as some women find relief from migraines while taking birth control pills while migraines can intensify for others.

Since hormone-based birth control can slightly increase the risk of blood clots, people experiencing migraine (especially with aura) should use caution as both birth control pills and migraines can slightly increase your risk of stroke. This may be remedied by taking pills not containing estrogen. The risk for a blood clot leading to stroke is higher in people who are overweight, have high blood pressure, smoke or are on bed rest for extended periods of time. Estrogen may also play a role through its effect on serotonin levels. If you find that your migraines tend to be associated with hormone changes, work with a qualified healthcare professional to balance your hormones. Using alternative methods for birth control is advised as you find a suitable birth control pill that works for you. Some of the other nutrients we have discussed, such as magnesium, may also help mitigate the effects of estrogen on migraines.

Therapies to Manage Symptoms of Migraine

Sometimes you just want something that makes you feel better while the migraine passes. To help manage the symptoms of migraine, try some of these natural remedies for relief. Each person experiences migraine a little differently, so experiment to find what works best for you. Hopefully, you will not need these very often if the other treatments have helped reduce your migraines.

Essential oils

Essential oils are naturally made by plants. They are extracted and distilled to create a highly concentrated product. Although the studies are small, some evidence suggests lavender and peppermint oil can be used to combat nausea, anxiety, sleeplessness and even some of the pain that comes with migraines. Try rubbing lavender on your wrists or neck. Put peppermint oil on your temples or back of your head or neck. Another option is to use topical rubs containing menthol. The cooling effect of these may be comforting in the early stages of a migraine attack. If smells bother you, this may not help. But if you can tolerate it, the oils or rubs may bring some relief. Be careful not to get too close to your eyes as it can cause a burning sensation. Used topically or in a diffuser, essential oils may help calm symptoms such as head pain or nausea. Experiment to see what works for you.

Ginger

The root of this Asian plant is often ingested to reduce nausea. It is available in supplement or tea form. One small study even indicated that ginger was as effective as sumatriptan to abort a migraine attack, without any adverse effects.[21] Ginger may not get rid of migraines completely, but it can help with some of the symptoms, like nausea.

Medical Cannabis and CBD Oil

After becoming legal in many states, medical marijuana, or cannabidiol (CBD), is an intriguing treatment option for many with migraine or cluster headache pain. Evidence is still preliminary, but promising.[22]

Thermal Therapy

Possibly one of the most popular natural remedies for migraine involves an ice pack. Cold therapy can be an effective form of acute self-care. The use of cold and heat together can also be beneficial to help alleviate pain associated with vascular changes. During a migraine attack, try putting your feet in hot water and a cold ice pack to the back of your neck or head (there are wearable ice packs or headache hats that help make this easier). This hot versus cold therapy causes vasoconstriction at the location of the ice pack and vasodilation at the feet. The object being to create vascular changes that relieve the pain from vasodilation in the brain and draw blood toward the feet. If you cannot place your feet in warm water, try placing your hands in warm water or under warm running water. This may be most helpful at the first sign of migraine.

Neuromodulation

Neuromodulation Devices (also known as stimulators) can be helpful in people that continue to have chronic migraine and for whom other therapy has not provided relief. This device sends magnetic waves or electric currents to your nervous system to help block the nerve impulses that cause pain. There are several types, including those that are implanted surgically and external ones that are handheld or wearable. Devices like this have been used to treat epilepsy and Parkinson's disease. Implanted units may need to be replaced over time and can lose effectiveness. The benefit should outweigh the risk of a surgical procedure. Another option is an FDA-approved external unit that works by stimulating the trigeminal nerve, which is believed to play a role in migraines. This unit (Cefaly®) is worn on your forehead with a sort of headband and sends pulses to the trigeminal nerve. It is lightweight so you can take it with you. These are only available with a doctor's prescription. This should be discussed with your neurologist to see if this would be an option for you, assuming other treatments or medications have already been exhausted.

———

Now that you are equipped with more information regarding possible migraine treatments, you can be your own advocate to get the best care possible. If any of the migraine triggers listed sound familiar and you believe one or more treatment methods may work for you, discuss these with your doctor. You are the most qualified to find which therapies or combinations work best for you. Keep in mind that most supplements and medications for migraine take a while (two to three months) to produce results. If you see no improvement in migraine symptoms, frequency, or duration within three months, try something else. In the next chapter, we will discuss how to talk to your doctor about migraines.

— 9 —
How to Talk to Your Doctor About Migraines

WHEN DEALING WITH a chronic condition like migraine, it is important to have a knowledgeable healthcare provider on your team. Having a support system in place, like friends and family, is crucial. There will be days when you cannot care for others or perform your regular activities. There may be days you cannot take care of yourself. Others you may include on your support team are your family doctor, neurologist, pharmacist, registered dietitian, massage therapist, counselor, chiropractor and acupuncturist. Surrounding yourself with people who are experts in their field can give you faster access to answers and treatment when you need it most.

In this chapter, we will discuss how you can prepare for a visit with your healthcare provider. We will explore questions to ask as well as information you can provide to give your doctor the information needed to treat you as the patient, not just a disease.

Things to Do Before Your Doctor Visit

There are things your doctor needs to know before being able to accurately diagnose and treat your migraines. You are the best source of information. Since there are no tests for migraine, the doctor will rely on information you provide to assess your condition and tailor a treatment that works best for you. To better equip you with that information, I recommend you keep a written record. A thorough history should include these four items.

Personal and Family Medical History

A personal and family medical history of migraine should include when your migraines started, any blood-related family members with migraine, identified triggers, associated symptoms, intensity of symptoms, how long they last, how frequently they occur and what you do to treat them.

Headache Log

Keeping a headache log will help you give better details. You should write down the date of migraine, what time it started, how long it lasted and any associated symptoms. It may also be helpful to include what you were doing before it started and what you had eaten within the past 24 hours. Add details such as intensity of pain, type of aura, or how you felt afterward. This can help you answer the doctor's questions better.

Food Log

If you have frequent headaches, it can be helpful to keep a diet diary or food log. This should include the date, times of meals and snacks, food eaten, beverages consumed, and any reactions observed to the food or beverages. Write down anything you put in your mouth throughout the day including candy and chewing gum. This can be of great value when trying to trace migraines to diet.

Medication and Treatment History

It is also beneficial for your doctor to know what treatments you have tried in the past. Include all medications whether over the counter or prescription and any supplements or herbal remedies. Make note of those that worked and those that did not. If you have tried other treatments such as massage or chiropractic care, share that with your healthcare provider.

Preparing for Your Doctor Visit

When you go for your doctor's visit, whether you are discussing a new onset of migraines, a long history of migraines or a change in your migraines, there are some questions your doctor may ask you.

1. Do you have a family history of migraines? Who and how are they related?

2. When did you first start having migraine? Did anything trigger the first migraine?

3. What symptoms do you have? How would you describe the pain? Do you get a warning signal before the headache begins? Does the pain gradually get worse or come on suddenly? Do you experience nausea and vomiting? Does anything aggravate your migraine?

4. How long do your migraines last? What is total time including migraine attack, initial symptoms beforehand and the "hangover" afterwards?

5. How many migraine attacks do you typically have per month?

6. What seems to help when you have a migraine? Other than medication, what do you do to get relief?

7. Have you noticed any food allergies or sensitivities associated with your migraines?

8. What other triggers have you noticed for migraines and do these always trigger a migraine?

9. Do they seem to occur at a certain time of day or month?

10. What medications, including prescription and over the counter, have you taken for migraine in the past? Which ones helped? Do you know the names and doses taken?

11. How often do you take medication to alleviate the pain?

12. Have you tried any other treatments such as massage, chiropractic, or acupuncture? Did anything help?

13. After the headache ends, do any symptoms hang around awhile? What type of symptoms and how long do they last?

14. Are you taking any prescribed or over the counter medications, supplements, or herbs on a regular basis?

15. Have you ever had a CT or MRI of your brain? If so, when?

16. Do you have any other medical conditions?

Be sure to describe in detail how migraine impacts your life. Does it keep you from being able to do your job? Have you missed family events or holiday gatherings because of migraine? Do you turn down opportunities because you are afraid migraine will keep you from being able to show up or perform your duties? Does it impact your family? The more you can describe the impact migraine has on your life, the better your doctor will understand how it affects you. Let them know how you feel about having migraines. Do migraines make you feel helpless, sad, depressed, frustrated, or angry? If your doctor has never experienced migraine, you may have to describe it in more detail for him or her. Do not be afraid to speak up to get the compassion and treatment that you deserve.

Remember that no one is more of an expert on your migraines than you are. You know your body, your symptoms, how you feel and how it impacts your life. Do not be intimidated by the doctor. He works for you and you are paying for help to find relief from a medical condition. If you do not feel heard or understood by your doctor, find another one. You need to feel comfortable talking to your healthcare provider and sharing your story. Do not hesitate to ask for a second opinion or referral to a specialist if you are not getting the results you desire. It is important to emphasize here that the goal for migraine treatment includes reduced frequency and intensity of migraine, not necessarily becoming migraine free. But you should see an improvement. The extent of improvement depends on your symptoms, history of diagnosis, complicating health conditions and previous treatments.

When to See a Specialist

Depending on the frequency and intensity of your headaches, your family doctor may be able to successfully treat your migraines. Some practitioners feel more comfortable treating headache disorders than others. A good time to ask for a referral to a specialist is if there is doubt about the diagnosis of your headaches, your attacks are getting worse or more frequent, or if you have not responded to treatments. When needed or upon your request, your doctor should always be willing to refer you to someone capable of providing the care you need.

A specialist will likely do a physical exam and ask about your migraines and medical history. Be prepared by knowing the answers to questions we discussed previously. He or she may also order some blood work or tests to rule out possible causes of migraine. This may take more than one visit. Figuring out migraine treatment can be a journey filled with some trial and error, so try to be patient. Remind yourself that the work involved can pay off with more migraine-free days.

What to Ask Your Doctor

Once your doctor has completed their assessment, they should have a better understanding of your condition. Learn as much as you can while you are with the doctor. Make sure he or she answers your questions. There is a lot of information to absorb and it can be hard to take everything in during one visit. It may help to take notes or bring a close friend or family member with you to the visit. Not only can they provide much-needed moral support, but they may hear things you miss and remember to ask questions you may have forgotten. Here are a few questions to ask your doctor.

1. What type of headaches do I have? If migraine, what type of migraine?

2. What medicines or treatment do you recommend for me? How often should these be taken?

3. What are some possible side effects of this medicine or treatment?

4. How long will it take for them to work?

5. How will I know the medicine is working?

6. What should I do if the medicines are not working?

7. Should I avoid any drugs because they might make my headaches worse?

8. Could non-drug treatments like massage, acupuncture or biofeedback help me?

9. What can I expect from my treatment plan? Will my migraines go away?

10. Are there any diet or lifestyle changes I can make?

11. Are there any tests I need?

12. When should I follow up with you again? Do I need another appointment, or can I just call you when needed?

Tips to Keep in Mind

For the best experience with your doctor visit, I recommend keeping a few things in mind.

1. Keep your answers brief and concise, but make sure to include important information. Your doctor has a busy schedule and needs to get the most information possible in a short amount of time. With that said, you still should not feel rushed during your appointment. You are paying the doctor to help you, but do not expect them to spend 30 or 45 minutes with you at each visit.

2. Keep a record! Having a written migraine history, headache log, diet diary, and medication list allows the doctor to skim through it to quickly find what he or she needs to know. This will improve their ability to diagnose and treat you.

3. Keep asking questions. If you do not feel you have gotten what you need, keep asking questions even if the doctor is ready to end your visit. If there is too much to cover, schedule a follow up visit to get your questions answered.

These tips should help you feel more confident when you go to see your doctor. For more information, I have included additional resources you may find helpful. Feel free to contact me if you have any questions. You will find my contact information on my website www.ourdailychews.com. Best wishes to you for migraine-free living!

ADDITIONAL RESOURCES

Get an electronic version of these resources here:

https://ourdailychews.com/overcoming-migraine-resources

Resources for More Information

American Headache Society

American Migraine Foundation

Association of Migraine Disorders

International Headache Society

Migraine Awareness Group

Migraine Research Foundation

National Headache Foundation

Support/Community Forums:

Migraine.com

Migraineagain.com

Find a headache specialist:

In the United States, check out the Find a Doctor tool under the resource section at https://americanmigrainefoundation.org/find-a-doctor/.

In the UK, check out https://www.migrainetrust.org/living-with-migraine/seeking-medical-advice/migraine-clinics/#clinic-map.

Supplements and Doses for Migraine Prevention

Supplement	Recommended Dose	Details
5-HTP	200 mg 2–3 times daily	400 to 600 mg used daily for migraine treatment in studies.
L-tryptophan	1 to 2 grams daily	May help with sleep. 2–4g daily has been used in migraine studies.
Melatonin	1 to 3 mg taken 30 minutes before bedtime	May help with sleep. Take as needed and start with lowest dose.
SAMe	400 to 800 mg twice daily	Research showed effective in treating depression and may help with inflammation.
Magnesium	300 to 400 mg daily in divided doses	Dose varies based on form of magnesium. Take with food. Get adequate calcium while taking magnesium.
Riboflavin	400 mg daily for 3 months	May work better when taken along with magnesium and CoQ10.
Folate	400 mcg daily	Easily acquired from fruits, vegetables, legumes and fortified foods.

Pyridoxine (B6)	1.3 to 1.7 mg daily	Meets the RDA for vitamin B6. Do not exceed 100 mg daily.
Cobalamin (B12)	400 to 500 mcg daily	Works with folic acid/folate.
Vitamin E	15 mg or 22 IU daily	A deficiency is rare. Avoid high doses as blood thinning can occur.
Vitamin C	500 mg daily	RDA is 75 mg for women and 90 mg for men, but it has been shown safe in higher doses.
CoQ10	150 to 300 mg daily	Research showed effective when taken for up to 3 months.
Butterbur	75 mg taken 1–2 times daily	Research showed effective when taken for up to 4 months.
Feverfew	50 to 150 mg once daily	Research showed effective when taken for up to 4 months.

Resources: https://naturalmedicines.therapeuticresearch.com/ and https://www.consumerlab.com/

Consult with a qualified healthcare provider before taking any supplement, especially if you have a health condition or are taking other medications.

Tools for Tracking Migraines

Try one of these apps to track your migraines:

iHeadache

Headache Log

Headache Tracker

Migraine Buddy

Migraine Headache Diary HeadApp

Migraine Insight

Migraine Monitor

N1-Headache

STOP Headache

Items to Include in Migraine Emergency Kit

Prescription or Over-the-counter Medications to Treat Attack

Bottle of Water

Nausea Medication or Ginger Chews/Candy

Ice Pack

Heat Pack

Essential Oil

Dark Sunglasses

Eye Mask

Earplugs or Cotton

Pillow

Blanket

Gallon-size Storage Bag (just in case)

Headphones and Player for Soothing Music

Acknowledgments

There are a few people without which this book would not have been possible. First, I want to thank my husband David for being supportive and understanding while I spent hours writing and editing this book. Thanks goes to my sister Tammy for always being an encourager. I also want to say thanks to Gary Williams and the amazing support group at Self-Publishing School for keeping me on track. And finally, my editor, Kim Carr at On The Mark Editorial Services, who deserves much credit for making this book readable.

About The Author

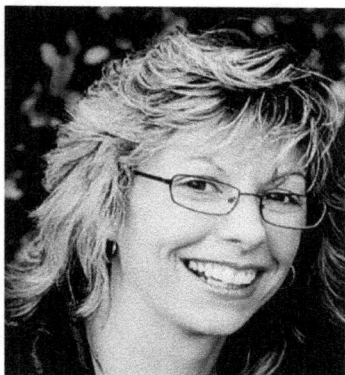

Lynn H. Clayton lives in North Carolina with her husband and two dogs. She is a private practice dietitian specializing in the management of diabetes and other chronic disease using medical nutrition therapy. Her interest has always been in the health field. She enjoys learning and helping people improve the quality of their lives. She began her professional career in the dental field as a registered dental hygienist. After seeing the impact diet has on oral health, she pursued a degree in nutrition. For over twelve years, she has worked in clinical and community nutrition promoting health by focusing on a healthy diet and lifestyle. After spending three decades on her personal journey to conquer migraines, the author felt compelled to share her knowledge with other migraineurs. Her hope is to help alleviate suffering for as many migraineurs as possible. By inspiring you toward improved quality of life using diet and lifestyle therapy, the author wants to give you the tools to overcome migraine.

When she is not seeing clients or writing, she enjoys spending time with her family, gardening, cooking, playing the piano and reading. For more information, visit her website at www.ourdailychews.com.

Can You Help?

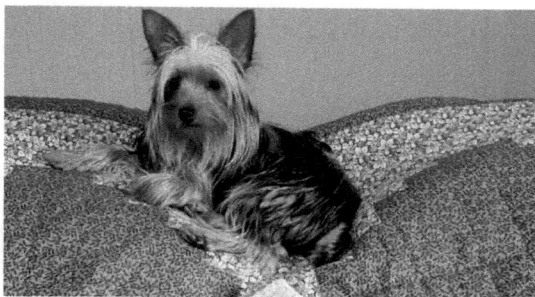

Thank You for Reading My Book!

I really appreciate your feedback, and I love hearing what you have to say.

I need your input to make the next version of this book and my future books better.

Please leave me an honest review on Amazon letting me know what you thought of the book.

Thanks so much!

Lynn H. Clayton

Notes

Chapter 1

[1] Historical overview. Migraine Awareness Group. Website. http://migraines.org/treatment/treathis.htm. Accessed April 15, 2020.

[2] Migraine history. Mandal, A MD. Medical.net. Website. *http://www.news-medical.net/health/Migraine-History.aspx*. Accessed May 15, 2020.

[3] Historical overview. Migraine Awareness Group. Website. http://migraines.org/treatment/treathis.htm. Accessed April 15, 2020.

[4] What is migraine. Migraine Research Foundation. Website. https://migraineresearchfoundation.org/about-migraine/what-is-migraine/. Accessed June 3, 2020.

[5] Headache and migraine diagnosis. Website. https://www.webmd.com/migraines-headaches/guide/making-diagnosis-doctors-exam#2. Published 2019. Accessed May 10, 2020.

[6] Life Extension Foundation for Longer Life. Migraine Headaches. In: Disease Prevention and Treatment. 5th edition. LE Publications, Inc. 2013:941.

[7] Migraine Headaches. Website. https://www.webmd.com/migraines-headaches/migraines-headaches-migraines. Reviewed May 23, 2018. Accessed June 3, 2020.

[8] 50 Famous people with migraine. Website. https://migrainepal. com/famous-with-migraine/. Published 2017. Accessed June 4, 2020.

[9] Steiner TJ, Stovner LJ, Birbeck GL. Migraine: the seventh disabler. *J Headache Pain*. 2013;14(1):1. Published 2013 Jan 10. doi:10.1186/1129-2377-14-1

[10] Migraine facts. Migraine Research Foundation. Website https:// migraineresearchfoundation.org/about-migraine/migraine-facts/. Accessed June 4, 2020.

Chapter 2

[1] Vickerstaff JJ. PhD, RD. Migraine and diet. In: The Health professional's guide to food allergies and intolerances. Chicago, IL. Academy of Nutrition and Dietetics; 2013:347.

[2] Sutherland HG, Albury CL, Griffiths LR. Advances in genetics of migraine. *J Headache Pain*. 2019;20(1):72. Published 2019 Jun 21. doi:10.1186/s10194-019-1017-9

[3] Migraine. Office on Women's Health. U.S. Department of Health and Human Services. https://www.womenshealth.gov/a-z-topics/migraine. Updated April 2019. Accessed May 29, 2020.

[4] Forty conditions associated with migraines. Website.https://www. migrainekey.com/blog/conditions-associated-with-migraines/. Accessed June 4, 2020.

[5] Migraine history. Mandal, A MD. Medical.net. Website. *http:// www.news-medical.net/health/Migraine-History.aspx*. Accessed April 15, 2020.

[6] Tfelt-Hansen, P, Koehler, P. History of the use of ergotamine and dihydroergotamine in migraine from 1906 and onward. Cephalalgia. 2008;28:877-886. doi:10.1111/j.1468-2982.2008.01578.x. Accessed June 10, 2020.

[7] Jacobs, B, Dussor, G. Neurovascular contributions to migraine: moving beyond vasodilation. Neuroscience. 2016; 338:130-144. www.ncbi.nlm.nih.gov/pubmed/27312704. Accessed June 19, 2020.

[8] Zhang X, Levy D, Noseda R, Kainz V, Jakubowski M, Burstein R. Activation of meningeal nociceptors by cortical spreading depression: implications for migraine with aura [published correction appears in J Neurosci. 2010 Jul 28;30(30):10259]. *J Neurosci*. 2010;30(26):8807-8814. doi:10.1523/ JNEUROSCI.0511-10.2010

[9] Enger R, Tang W, Vindedal G F, Jensen V, Helm P J, Sprengel R, Looger L L, Nagelhus E A. Dynamics of ionic shifts in cortical spreading depression. *Cereb Cortex*. 2015; 25 (11): 4469-4476. www.ncbi.nlm.nih.gov/pmc/articles/PMC4816793. Accessed June 19, 2020.

[10] Caspary, E, Comaish, J. Release of serotonin from human platelets in hypersensitivity states. Nature. 1967; 214, 286–287. https:// doi.org/10.1038/214286a0. Accessed June 19, 2020.

[11] Migraine phases. Robert, T. Website. https://migraine.com/ migraine-basics/migraine-phases/. Published 2011. Accessed June 4, 2020.

[12] Scher AI, Launer LJ. Migraine: migraine with aura increases the risk of stroke. Nat Rev Neurol. 2010;6(3):128-129. doi:10.1038/ nrneurol.2010.14.

[13] Migraines and the link to other health conditions. Website. https://www.webmd.com/migraines-headaches/can- migraines-lead-to-other-health-conditions.Reviewed 2019. Accessed June 12, 2020.

[14] Migraine triggers and how to deal with them. Website. https:// americanmigrainefoundation.org/resource-library/top-10- migraine-triggers-and-how-to-deal-with-them/. Accessed June 10, 2020.

Chapter 3

[1] Dietary reference intakes for water, potassium, sodium, chloride and sulfate. Food and Nutrition Board of the National Institutes of Health. https://www.nal.usda.gov/sites/default/files/fnic_ uploads/water_full_report.pdf. Accessed May 30, 2020.

Chapter 5

[1] Triggers of migraine. Association of Migraine Disorders. Website. https://www.migrainedisorders.org/migraine-disorders/ triggers/. Accessed June 12, 2020.

Chapter 6

[1] Monro J, Carini C, Brostoff J, Zilkha K. *Food allergy in migraine: study of dietary exclusion and RAST. Lancet, 1980;2(8184):1-4.*

[2] Migraine and diet. In: Vickerstaff Joneja J. The Health Professional's Guide to Food Allergies and Intolerances. Chicago, IL. Academy of Nutrition and Dietetics; 2013:347.

[3] Monro J, Carini C, Brostoff J, Zilkha K. *Food allergy in migraine: study of dietary exclusion and RAST. Lancet, 1980;2(8184):1-4.*

[4] Migraine and diet. In: Vickerstaff Joneja J. The Health Professional's Guide to Food Allergies and Intolerances. Chicago, IL. Academy of Nutrition and Dietetics; 2013:348.

[5] Migraine and diet. In: Vickerstaff Joneja J.The Health Professional's Guide to Food Allergies and Intolerances. Chicago, IL. Academy of Nutrition and Dietetics; 2013:349.

[6] Purves D, Augustine GJ, Fitzpatrick D, et al., eds. The biogenic amines. In: Neuroscience. 2nd ed. Sunderland, MA: Sinauer Associates; 2001. Accessed at https://www.ncbi.nlm.nih.gov/ books/NBK11035/

[7] Migraine and diet. In: Vickerstaff Joneja J.The Health Professional's Guide to Food Allergies and Intolerances. Chicago, IL. Academy of Nutrition and Dietetics; 2013:349.

[8] Migraine and diet. In: Vickerstaff Joneja J.The Health Professional's Guide to Food Allergies and Intolerances. Chicago, IL. Academy of Nutrition and Dietetics; 2013:350.

[9] Migraine and diet. In: Vickerstaff Joneja J.The Health Professional's Guide to Food Allergies and Intolerances. Chicago, IL. Academy of Nutrition and Dietetics; 2013:351.

[10] Elimination Diets. In: Vickerstaff Joneja J.The Health Professional's Guide to Food Allergies and Intolerances. Chicago, IL. Academy of Nutrition and Dietetics; 2013:81.

[11] Helfand M, Peterson K. Drug class review: triptans: final report update 4. Portland, OR. Oregon Health & Science University. 2009. https://www.ncbi.nlm.nih.gov/books/NBK47282/.

Chapter 7

[1] Tepper D. Calcitonin gene-related peptide targeted therapy for migraine. Website. https://americanmigrainefoundation.org/resource-library/calcitonin-gene-related-peptide-targeted-therapy-migraine/. Published 2016. Accessed May 27, 2020.

[2] Young, S N. J Psychiatry Neuroscience. 2007; 32(6):394-399. https://www.ncbi.nlm.nih.gov/pmc/articles/PMC2077351/. Accessed June 19, 2020.

Chapter 8

[1] Sicuteri F. The ingestion of serotonin precursors (L-5-Hydroxytryptophan and L-tryptophan) improves migraine headache. Headache. 1973;13(1):19-22.

[2] Life Extension Foundation for Longer Life. Migraine headaches. In: Disease Prevention and Treatment. 5th edition. United States. LE Publications, Inc. 2013:945.

[3] Long R, Zhu Y, Zhou S. Therapeutic role of melatonin in migraine prophylaxis: A systematic review. *Medicine (Baltimore)*. 2019;98(3):e14099. doi:10.1097/MD.0000000000014099

[4] Life Extension Foundation for Longer Life. Migraine Headaches. In: Disease Prevention and Treatment. 5th edition. United States. LE Publications, Inc. 2013:945.

[5] Peikert A, Wilmzig C, Kohne-Volland R. Prophylaxis of migraine with oral magnesium: results from a prospective, multi-center, placebo-controlled and double-blind randomized study. Cephalalgia. 1996;16:257–63.

6 Dietary reference intake for magnesium. https://ods.od.nih.gov/factsheets/Magnesium-HealthProfessional/. Accessed June 19, 2020.

7 Peikert A, Wilimzig C, Köhne-Volland R. Prophylaxis of migraine with oral magnesium: results from a prospective, multicenter, placebo-controlled and double-blind randomized study. *Cephalalgia*. 1996;16(4):257-263. doi:10.1046/j.1468-2982.1996.1604257.x

8 Köseoglu E, Talaslioglu A, Gönül AS, Kula M. The effects of magnesium prophylaxis in migraine without aura. *Magnes Res*. 2008;21(2):101-108.

9 Fischbach F. A Manual of Laboratory and Diagnostic Tests. 7th ed. United States of America. Lippincott Williams & Wilkins. 2004;961.

10 Shaik M, Hua Gan, S. Vitamin supplementation as possible prophylactic treatment against migraine with aura and menstrual migraine. Biomed Res Int. 2015: 469529. Published online 2015 Feb 28. doi: 10.1155/2015/469529. Accessed May 30, 2020.

11 Sun-Edelstein C, Mauskop A. Alternative headache treatments: nutraceuticals, behavioral and physical treatments. Headache. 2011 Feb;51(3):469-483. https://doi.org/10.1111/j.1526-4610.2011.01846.x.

12 Folate fact sheet for health professionals. https://ods.od.nih.gov/factsheets/Folate-HealthProfessional/. Last updated June 3, 2020. Accessed June 19, 2020.

13 Vitamin E fact sheet for health professionals. https://ods.od.nih.gov/factsheets/VitaminE-HealthProfessional/. Last updated February 28, 2020. Accessed June 19, 2020.

14 Vitamin C fact sheet for healthcare professionals. https://ods.od.nih.gov/factsheets/VitaminC-HealthProfessional/. Last updated February 27, 2020. Accessed June 19, 2020.

[15] Sun-Edelstein C, Mauskop A. Alternative headache treatments: nutraceuticals, behavioral and physical treatments. Headache. 2011 Feb;51(3):469-483. https://doi.org/10.1111/j.1526-4610.2011.01846.x.

[16] Coenzyme Q10. Website. https://migraine.com/migraine-treatment/natural-remedies/coenzyme-q10/. Published November 29, 2010. Accessed June 8, 2020.

[17] Sun-Edelstein C, Mauskop A. Alternative headache treatments: nutraceuticals, behavioral and physical treatments. Headache. 2011 Feb;51(3):469-483. https://doi.org/10.1111/j.1526-4610.2011.01846.x.

[18] Sun-Edelstein C, Mauskop A. Alternative headache treatments: nutraceuticals, behavioral and physical treatments. Headache. 2011 Feb;51(3):469-483. https://doi.org/10.1111/j.1526-4610.2011.01846.x.

[19] Edlow AG, Bartz D. Hormonal contraceptive options for women with headache: a review of the evidence. *Rev Obstet Gynecol.* 2010;3(2):55-65.https://www.ncbi.nlm.nih.gov/pmc/articles/PMC2938905/. Accessed June 22, 2020.

[20] Maghbooli, M., F. Golipour, A. Moghimi, and M. Yousefi. Comparison between the efficacy of ginger and sumatriptan in the ablative treatment of the common migraine. Phytotherapy Research: PTR. U.S. National Library of Medicine. 2014. Web. 02 Jan. 2018.

[21] Glaser, A. Cannabis relieves migraine pain by nearly half, study says. Website. www.migraineagain.com. Published 2019. Accessed June 22, 2020.

[22] Rodriguez, T. Epilepsy and migraine: a common ground? Website. https://www.neurologyadvisor.com/topics/epilepsy/epilepsy-and-migraine-a-common-ground/. Published 2015. Accessed June 12, 2020.